Invisible Men

Finding, Engaging, and Inspiring Men in Therapy

Invisible Men

Finding, Engaging, and Inspiring Men in Therapy

David Grove, LISW

with

Rhonda Burnaugh

Zeig, Tucker & Theisen, Inc.
Phoenix, Arizona

Library of Congress Cataloging-in-Publication Data
Grove, David, 1956–
Invisible men : finding, engaging, and inspiring men in therapy / David Grove with Rhonda Burnaugh.
p. cm.
Includes bibliographical references.
ISBN 1-891944-95-9 (alk. paper)
1. Men — Mental health. 2. Men — Psychology. 3. Family psychotherapy. I. Burnaugh, Rhonda. II. Title.

RC451.4.M45 G76 2002
616.89'156--dc21 2002016754

Published by

ZEIG, TUCKER & THEISEN, INC.
3614 North 24th Street
Phoenix, AZ 85016

Manufactured in the United States of America

10 9 8 7 6 5 4 3 2 1

To Our Fathers:

David

Gere

Bud

and

Butch

Table of Contents

Acknowledgments

This book was inspired by a series of conversations among Jay Haley, Neil Schiff, Rhonda Burnaugh, and the author that took place in Jay Haley's home from 1993 to 1995. The group would meet for several hours every few months to share cases. Initially, the purpose was to organize a casebook demonstrating ways to help seriously disturbed clients. We took turns offering cases, examining outcomes, and describing what seemed to help when we were successful. As the discussions unfolded, an interesting phenomenon became apparent. No matter who the identified patient was, a young adult, an adolescent, or a married woman, there always seemed to be a man in the background making a significant but not readily apparent contribution to the problem. In case after case, the success of the outcome seemed dependant on involving this man in the therapy. Either how he was responding to the client presenting with the problem had to be drastically changed, or he had to be helped with a serious problem of his own in order to help the client improve significantly. The group disbanded when Haley moved to California and the idea of organizing a casebook lost its appeal. Nevertheless, what was obvious was that a book about passive men was in order.

For years prior to the group meetings, Neil Schiff had been observing the phenomenon on his own and had called attention to it, even giving workshops on the topic. Dr. Schiff, therefore, deserves much of the credit for the idea. The therapy approach presented in the book is Strategic Family Therapy, and Haley gets obvious credit for influencing the way in which the cases are described and dealt with. Two of the cases, "Married with No Children" and "A First Child," were actually presented in the group. "A Powerful Daughter" is a case on which I had consulted with Haley before the group began to meet. In these three cases, Haley and the group share credit for the way in which the cases were viewed and the interventions devised.

Although most of the cases presented here are from my own practice, several are from the caseloads of therapists with whom I have consulted. I would like to thank those therapists for allowing me to include their work: Dale McClure and Eugene Bell.

Rhonda Burnaugh is listed as a co-author due to her extensive participation in making this book a reality. She is offering one case, "Married with No Children," in detail, and also contributed several other case examples throughout this book. In addition to participating in the group meetings, she acted as an editor and critic throughout the process of writing this book. Her major contribution, however, was the inspiration for the project. At the time the group decided to meet, Rhonda was the nurse for the medical director of a major clinic. She had won his trust and so could choose cases on which she wished to work and was in charge of how to do it. Without the relationship she had with the doctor, we never would have had the opportunity to work the way we did with several of the cases presented in this book. She suggested that we involve Jay Haley in discussions about the cases, most of which related to psychotic clients. I proposed the idea to Haley and suggested that Neil Schiff be included in the group. A project was born.

Finally, I would like to acknowledge three colleagues who encouraged me to write the book, reviewed parts or all of it, and offered support when it appeared that the project was in jeopardy: Jim Lantz, Pat Early, and Gilbert Greene.

David Grove

Foreword by Jay Haley

It is always interesting to find a new idea blossoming in Family Therapy. It shows the richness of its content. In exploring the ideas presented in "Invisible Men" (what a nice title) one will encounter both a newness and a tradition.

I recall the 1950s and the effort to understand the organizational sequences of a family when we had only the language of individual therapy as a descriptor. Ultimately, we came out with at least one sequence and one family structure. It may have been the first concept of its kind in the field of Family Therapy. We began to understand the problem as unfolding in steps, or sequences:

Step 1: A child manifested a problem and a therapist was brought in. The therapist dealt with the child individually, actually playing with him or her.

Step 2: When that intervention failed, the therapist brought in the child's mother and the mother and child were focused on as a dyad, with the mother being taught to parent.

Step 3: When that intervention failed, the therapist brought the father in and asked him to take charge. In those days, he was called "the peripheral father."

Step 4: When the father began to deal with the child, the mother would get into conflict with father, objecting to how he was dealing with the child, among other things.

Step 5: The mother and father were helped to resolve their conflicts while talking about the child, and the child then no longer expressed a problem.

For the contemporary scene, this book by David Grove manifests all the coalitions and variations in an organization that a family can devise. Husband and wife are dealt with, as are mother and daughter, as are son and mother, and let's not neglect stepmother and what of stepfather? The common theme throughout is a peripheral man causing, or unable to avoid, family conflicts. If mother and daughter go after each other, father disappears. Problems then escalate. One implication of this survey of our field is that feminists need to develop ways of helping men to be more manly, since it would appear that that is what women prefer men to be.

How much more complex and interesting are the variations of men's involvement with their families as compared with the simple peripheral father back in that revolutionary decade of the 1950s.

Foreword by Neil Schiff

In the early 1980s, Cloe Madanes, one of the co-directors of the Family Therapy Institute of Washington, D.C., observed offhandedly that in many of the couples and families that came to the Institute for treatment, the husband's socioeconomic background was of lower status than that of the wife's. This comment stuck with me and led me to think more extensively in general about the role and functioning of the husband and/or father in the family. Family therapy has long focused on triangles in the family, at least since the 1950s when it was discovered, as Jay Haley wrote, "that schizophrenics had fathers," which coincided with the shift in thinking from dyads to triads. Family therapy formulated one widely taught paradigm of family functioning: when a child was presented as a problem, that involved a so-called peripheral father whose symptomatic child's problem was construed as an attempt to involve the father more in the family. As I thought more critically about the man in the family, I began to realize that in one case after another, the man was not simply peripheral but impaired, and that one way of thinking about the presenting problem was that it represented an opportunity for the man to recover his ability to function, which, once accomplished, usually led to an improvement in the presenting problem. I recognized that a useful way of thinking about therapy was that it was mostly about men. Even in situations like the typical triangle involving a mother, grandmother, and troubled child, there was often a man, usually in the background or invisible (to use David Grove's apt term), whose impaired functioning contributed to the presenting problem. If the therapist attended to this phenomenon, it made a case more intelligible and led to more effective interventions.

I began to teach supervisees the utility of this idea and referred to cases in which the idea was explanatory and helpful such as, "make my husband a mensh" cases, mensh being a Yiddish word that means, "a human being; an upright, honorable, decent person; someone of consequence," according to the definition in Leo Rosten's *Joy of Yiddish*. In workshops on strategic therapy where parsing videotaped cases was part of the instructional method, the relevance of the idea became clear to attendees irrespective of whether the case presented as a child problem, an out-of-control adolescent or young adult problem, a marital problem, or something else. In fact, it appeared that the true secret of psychotherapy, if there was one, was again that it was useful to think about therapy as mostly helping impaired men, whether or not they were even in the treatment room.

Unsurprisingly, when the project, initiated and described herein by David Grove, began in 1993, the idea of impaired men explained more and more of what was going on in the families we discussed, independent of the presenting problem. In 1996, David Grove arranged for me to give a workshop at Ohio State (generously cosponsored by the university's School of Social Work) which he attended and where he too observed again in a selection of apparently different and difficult cases how this idea explained so much in the way of problems and led to useful ideas about how to intervene. He proposed that the idea provided a framework for making sense of and resolving the many different problems presented to therapists, including, particularly, the collection of refractory cases we had all conversed about over the course of the two years (1993–1995) when we met.

To his great credit, David Grove developed and elaborated this idea as an organizing and explanatory framework in this book about therapy with extremely difficult problems that follows. In a series of diverse and remarkable cases, seen by him and his wife, Rhonda Burnaugh, and deconstructed herein, he demonstrates the application of the idea of invisible men to thinking about cases and the use of the idea in generating interventions that resolve the presenting problems.

I admire David Grove's enthusiasm, determination, and hard work. This book gestated in his thinking for years and went through numerous iterations before it assumed its present form. David Grove has a way of writing that is easy to read, engaging, and often dramatic. He brings the reader into the client's and therapist's world, illustrating the idea of invisible men and using the idea as an explanation, as well as a basis for change.

Introduction

A 12-year-old girl lived with her father and stepmother. The family came to the attention of child protective services when it was reported that the stepmother was emotionally abusive to her stepdaughter. After protective services investigated the family, an in-home therapist was assigned to the case to try to help avoid placing the girl in foster care.

On his first visit with the family, the therapist interviewed the stepmother and her husband. During the interview, the stepmother behaved bizarrely, and was extremely hostile toward the girl. When discussing her with the therapist, the stepmother became wildly and intensely angry, and indirectly threatened the girl. At one point, she leaned toward the therapist and while clenching her fists, looked at him with wild eyes, and cited a list of the girl's petty offenses, referring to her as "that fucking bitch." Despite his patience and attempts to empathize with the woman, the therapist could not have a reasonable interview with her. When asked about basic facts concerning the girl, the woman's face became red, her body began to shake uncontrollably, and her voice trembled with anger. The therapist was taken aback by the stepmother's irrational behavior. His attempts to connect with her and to include the husband in the conversation failed. The husband sat quietly during the entire bizarre scene and only responded to the therapist with one-word answers.

The therapist learned that the daughter had been living with the couple for less than a year. Prior to that, she had been in foster care after being removed from her biological mother's home. The girl had had a tumultuous year and now was living with a very angry stepmother and a father who did not stand up for his daughter, but would withdraw both emotionally and physically by leaving the home and going out with his male friends.

After his initial interview, the therapist had three successive interviews that were replicas of the first. He was very concerned about the girl, who bore the brunt of her stepmother's terrible anger. The stepmother's behavior and angry pronouncements about the child were approaching psychotic dimensions.

After his fourth interview with the family, the therapist consulted with the author about the case. It was becoming clear that if nothing changed, the girl might again be removed from the home by protective services, an intervention that the therapist wanted to avoid, although he was very pessimistic about the situation. He described the woman as out of her mind and in need of heavy medication.

To try to get beyond the impasse, it was suggested that the therapist intervene with the *father*. The plan was for the therapist to meet with the father privately and to make an all-out effort to get him more engaged with the family. One possibility was for the father to take a strong stand with his wife and insist that she stop treating the girl so badly. But, considering the situation, it was decided not to go in this direction. Instead, the father would be urged to be more attentive and nurturing to his wife.

The therapist then launched a major effort to join with the father, persuading him to do his utmost to treat his wife positively and more affectionately. Over the next two weeks, the therapist met with the father individually on four occasions and coached the man on wooing his wife. To the therapist's amazement, the result was an almost miraculous turnaround. As the man began to treat his wife better, she in turn began to soften toward the daughter. A woman whose upset was approaching psychotic proportions changed dramatically when the therapist intervened with the *husband* individually. After the therapy strategy had been determined, the stepmother did not even take part in the interviews! As the case unfolded, more details emerged explaining how the family got into this situation and why the stepmother was in such turmoil, but the basic strategy was maintained. The husband was put in charge of helping his wife chill out. What happened here? Why did this intervention work? Perhaps another case can provide some answers.

Twenty-three-year-old John paid an afternoon visit to his parents, who led isolated lives in a rural community. His father, a very soft-spoken, unassuming man, was retired and his mother was in poor health. John was the only one of their three children who lived in the area and saw them on a regular basis. But, although often lonely, John's parents did not express gratitude for their son's attention. He was said to be schizophrenic and was very skilled at antagonizing his mother, although she was the one who threw irrational fits of ranting and raving. On this particular afternoon, John had just come from his aunt's home, which he also visited regularly. It seemed he enjoyed stirring the family pot and getting his mother and aunt worked up and on the phone with one another. Typically, they did not speak with each other unless John had provoked them.

A few minutes into this latest visit with his parents, John asked his mother if she had been to her sister's home recently and had seen the sister's pond. When she said that she had not, John told her coolly that she was missing something. There were dismembered human body parts floating in it. The mother erupted, accusing John of trying to cause her to have a heart attack. She stormed around the house flailing her arms and carrying on, while John laughed and continued to interject graphic descriptions of floating body parts between her howls. The scene was both comical and unnerving. Finally, the mother insisted that John leave and not come back. Having had his fun, John departed while continuing to mock his mother.

Three days later, John visited again and behaved very well. He did not try to antagonize his mother, even though she was still upset and he could easily have done so. Nevertheless, the damage had been done.

A therapist attempting to intervene here would have several

options. One could focus on the son, and attempt to restrain him from antagonizing his mother, either by insisting he take additional medication or by trying some other approach. One could also focus on the mother, attempting to help her not to be so reactive, or to take some proactive initiative that would prevent the entire episode. One could ask the mother to think of times when her son did not provoke her, and to try to act as she had on those occasions. A therapist seeing the two of them together and witnessing such an episode would be hard pressed to stay out of the struggle. The mother and son together could be the focus of the intervention, and suggestions could be offered to the two of them. What I am suggesting is to do none of the above.

Intervening with either the mother or son individually, or with the two together, would mean missing a crucial aspect of this interchange. The absent party in either scenario would be the father. He was rendered invisible by the intensity and extreme irrationality of his wife and son.

One can imagine his dilemma. He may have been reluctant to intervene, fearing he might escalate the outbreak. He may just have wanted peace and knew from experience that they both would calm down eventually if he stayed out of it. It could be that it was against his nature to become involved in such an uproar. In any case, he was guilty of the sin of omission and this was a major contributing factor in the upheaval. By remaining silent while his son antagonized his wife, he was essentially siding with his son. By not taking a stand, he was communicating his tolerance of the son's behavior. When his son returned the next day, he again passively sided with his son by not insisting that the son leave. Even though John was well-behaved, his mother had clearly indicated that he was not welcome. By not berating John for returning against his mother's wishes, the father was again siding with his son against his wife. The father was in a cross-generational coalition with his son against his wife, a fact that was concealed by the father's passivity (Haley, 1967).

A therapist choosing to leave this father out of an intervention would be guilty of the same sin of omission as the father. By not including the father, a therapist would be communicating tolerance of the father's passivity, implying that only the wife and/or son needed to change. The wife would then be in the dilemma of cooperating with a therapy that did not include her husband. And the very act of her participating in a therapy that left her husband out would imply her agreement with the view that her husband did not need to change.

When faced with some serious problem in his family, a man can respond in either of two extreme ways that will exacerbate the problem. If his son is out of control, he can overreact and become violent, or he can under react and do nothing, responding with passivity. What might be helpful would be for him to make his presence felt, without doing anything extreme.

Of these two extremes, it is the passive one that will be the focus of this book. We are arguing that, in some instances, sins of omission are far more destructive than are sins of overreaction. Passive behavior by a man when some action is required can be disastrous.

This is a book about men who do not act when action is desperately needed. It is about men whose teenage daughters spray-paint "fuck" on the walls of the house, or commandeer the family van and drive to another region of the country. It is about men whose wives have quit their jobs and stay at home, dragging themselves around the house as if they were dying, or binge and purge almost to the point of death, or aimlessly wander around the neighborhood at 2:00 A.M., covered in dog's blood. But while their wives and children are behaving in these extreme ways, the men calmly sit and read the paper, or play golf, or flip through the television channels on the remote. At the office, these same men may aggressively pursue careers that require them to assert themselves if they are to be successful. Although they are not passive when at work, in their homes, they have become invisible. The problem is occurring within the family context. Why do they act in this dual way and what can be done about it? Intervening with these men often means intervening in their intimate relationships. This book is about how to understand the problem from an interactional perspective, engage men in treatment, and motivate them to take action.

1

Contract for Invisibility

QUID PRO QUO

One way to approach the problem of men disappearing at home is to view the issue as part of a relationship contract. The idea that couples follow rules, or a contract, which are implicitly worked out was first proposed by Don Jackson (Jackson, 1965; Lederer & Jackson, 1968). Jackson's concept of quid pro quo was not limited to married couples. Jackson argued that it can apply to any two people engaged in a long-term relationship, including gay couples, and even couples who are still following an established pattern after they have divorced. Although many examples in this book are of married couples, when a man disappears within the context of a relationship, that relationship does not have to be a marriage.

According to Jackson, couples negotiate implicitly over time through their behavioral responses to each other regarding various issues. If, for example, the husband turns the thermostat down to 72 degrees and the wife does not make an issue of it, they have compromised regarding the temperature, with no words spoken. Jackson argued that most issues in a long-term relationship are negotiated in this implicit manner.

An important point here is that the couples are not negotiating verbally. Three concepts allow for implicit negotiating (Watzlawick, Bavelas, & Jackson, 1967; Jackson, 1961). The first is the

Bateson idea that every verbal communication is simultaneously both a report and a command. The communicant is simultaneously reporting information and implicitly issuing a command. How the respondent reacts to the implicit command then clarifies the nature of the two participants' relationship. Second is the idea that all behavior is communication. One cannot avoid sending and responding to messages. Third is that the context in which the message is being communicated clarifies the meaning of the communication.

For example, suppose a wife announces to her husband, "It is trash day." She is not just offering information, but could also be implying that she wants her husband to take out the trash. She is assigning a task. Only someone in authority can assign a task and, therefore, she is asserting herself as in a position of authority in relation to her husband. How the husband responds to this statement then clarifies their relationship, if she really has the authority to assign him a task. If he responds by taking out the trash, he is communicating that he will cooperate if she gives him a task, and thus, at least in the area of housework, the wife can assign tasks to the husband. They did not discuss the issue verbally. It was decided by how the husband responded behaviorally to the wife's implicit command that he take out the trash.

What if the husband does not agree that his wife should have authority over him regarding the housework? Suppose the wife feels she is doing more than her share of housework, and it is in this context that she says, "It is trash day." Suppose also that the husband reacts differently to being given an order by his wife. He may not agree that she should have the authority to delegate household tasks. He might interpret it to mean that she is in charge of the house. The issue is not about the particular item of who should take out the trash, it is whether or not the wife has the power to give an order and delegate chores. Suppose she already is in charge of the paychecks, which are deposited in an account that she handles, and she already is in charge of how to deal with the children. If she is also in charge of the house, she is in charge of everything, and this is not an equal relationship. But the husband does not comment on the fact that she is delegating chores, or that he feels one down in two other major areas of their life. Instead, he says he does all of the outside work, and he does not think it is his job to do inside work. She responds by angrily listing 27 more chores that she does than he does. The husband, reacting to the intensity of his wife's response, backs down and takes out the trash.

In this example, the disagreement was on a process level, namely, that the husband did not agree that the wife had the authority to delegate household tasks in an overall context in which she already had authority over the money and the children. None of these issues, however, were discussed. The discussion occurred in response to one specific issue, and spilled over into who does the most chores. Although disagreement was on a process level, it was discussed on a content level. Second, the husband withdrew from the discussion to avoid the intensity of his wife's reaction. He capitulated, but he did not agree. The couple did not resolve the issue to the satisfaction of both parties, a process that would have defined them as equals. To do this, the wife would have to be willing to listen to the husband, and the husband would have to be willing to state his case. Instead, the wife became upset and the husband capitulated. Both played a part in bringing verbal negotiations to a halt.

On a process level, the husband was left in a one-down position in the marriage, in the sense that his wife was in charge of the house, the money, and the children. It would appear that the spouses did not share equal power, with the wife the more powerful partner. Further, with this couple, it was unlikely that power would be equalized by verbal negotiations. They had a pattern in which the wife strongly asserted herself and the husband, even though he did not agree, capitulated in order to avoid his wife's intense reaction to his disagreeing.

Jackson argued, however, that in all long-term relationships, power is always equal. He argued that in the situation described above, the supposed one-down spouse would equalize power in some indirect way, if it could not be equalized overtly through open negotiations. If the husband cannot take on his wife verbally, one way in which he can equalize the relationship is by passively resisting. He might develop a bad back and be unable to do chores. Or he might work all the time and never be available to do them. Or he might procrastinate and not get his chores done until the wife becomes exasperated and does them herself. If he responds in any of these ways, he has equalized the situation by not following her command, but he has accomplished this at the expense of his status. He has equalized power by lowering his status. A bad back means he cannot function physically. Working all the time means he is neglecting his family. Procrastinating means he cannot be counted on to do the simplest chore. In all of these scenarios, he has cut his wife down to size by lowering himself.

The wife may suspect that he is upset and ask him if he is angry about something. He may fear that if he says he thinks the situation is unfair, his wife will become upset. To avoid this possibility, he answers, "Everything is fine."

In this example, we have several of the ingredients in the recipe for making a man invisible. First, we have partners who do not agree on a larger issue, such as who has authority in what situation. Next, they do not discuss the disagreement on the level on which it is occurring, but fight about a particular item, not understanding that how that item is resolved sets a precedence in a larger context. Third, we have a wife who becomes intensely upset about the disagreement and a husband who withdraws from the argument by capitulating. He is not agreeing with his wife, he is backing down to appease her and to avoid the intensity of her reaction. Because this leaves him in an unequal position in the marriage, he equalizes the relationship in a passive, indirect way, which results in some loss of status for him. A man who works all of the time is invisible at home. A man who capitulates all of the time is invisible in the sense that it is unclear what he really believes. The partners develop a contract, a quid pro quo, where the wife can give orders and the husband will accept, but will passively equalize the relationship at his own reputation's expense.

The Psychology of Uncertainty

What happens when a husband says one thing and does another?

What is his wife to think when he verbally agrees to do more around the house, but behaviorally always manages not to? He is sending his wife a double message, creating an uncertainty about what he really thinks. This is one thing when the issue is a minor one, such as a household chore, but takes on a much greater magnitude when the issue is something like whether or not the husband really wants them to have a baby, or if he still finds his wife attractive or still loves her, or if he prefers his daughter's company to that of his wife's.

In addition to an inability to negotiate, another possibility that can result in a man's vanishing is that he is ambivalent about something. It is not that he and his wife have a disagreement that is not being discussed openly, but that the husband is uncertain about something and this is not being discussed. Whatever the issue, he himself is uncertain and is struggling with how he really does feel. In either case, if the husband is avoiding conflict with his wife, and just telling her what he thinks she wants to hear in relation to issues of this magnitude, real problems may develop.

If the husband is sending double messages and the wife is uncertain regarding his feelings on an important issue, there will be tension in the relationship until the husband clarifies his position. The problem is that if he is stating what he thinks his wife wants to hear, then his saying something is not going to satisfy his wife. Behavioral communication is required. When faced with someone who says one thing and does another, actions speak louder than words. To clarify how he really feels, an ambivalent husband has to back up his words with actions. More specifically, if he is saying what his wife wants to hear, he is responding verbally to an inquiry that she is initiating. She might ask, "Do you really want this baby?" He then responds, "Of course I do." Part of the pattern is that she initiates and he responds. He does not initiate behavior on his own as a signal that would clarify his position. He does not initiate behavior spontaneously.

It is assumed here that spontaneous behavior is the ultimate indicator of where an individual stands on any given issue. If a husband is attracted to his wife, his eyes light up when she enters the room. If he loves her, he initiates affection. If his wife is pregnant and he is excited about her having a baby, he will take actions that indicate his excitement. It is his spontaneous initiatives, not his verbal responses to inquiries, that clarify his feelings.

If the partners are in a pattern, however, in which the wife makes a demand and the husband capitulates in order to avoid conflict, the pattern is one in which the wife initiates and the husband responds to the wife's initiative. The husband does not initiate anything. His spontaneous initiatives are regulated by this pattern. The wife may insist on having a baby and the husband goes along. They are following their pattern. But if the husband shows no spontaneous behavior that demonstrates that he truly wants a child, the wife is going to become uncertain. She may then ask, "Do you really want this child?" He, of course, says he does. This response will not clarify his position because he is just following their pattern. Only his spontaneous action will clarify his position, but his initiation of spontaneous behavior is the very thing their pattern does not allow.

When partners develop a pattern in which the husband agrees to everything, invariably the wife will be left uncertain. Two examples come from *Pragmatics of Human Communication* (Watzlawick, Bavelas, & Jackson, 1967).

Example 1:

PSYCHIATRIST: You are saying that you don't get clues from your husband that you need to let you know if he likes what you are doing?

WIFE: Yes.

PSYCHIATRIST: Does he criticize you?

WIFE: Rarely does he criticize. He compliments you. You see, that is the befuddling thing. Suppose I cook something and I burn it. He says it's really "very, very nice." Then, if I make something that is extra nice, it is "very, very nice." I told him I don't know whether something is nice — I don't know whether he is criticizing me or complimenting me. . . .

PSYCHIATRIST: So you really don't know where you stand with someone who always compliments.

WIFE: No, I don't know whether he is criticizing me or really sincerely complimenting me.

In this example, the husband is patronizing his wife. No matter what she does, he compliments her. He does not say what he really thinks. In this sense, he is invisible and his disappearance makes his wife uncertain.

Example 2:

HUSBAND (to therapist): From long experience I know that if I want peace at home I must not interfere with the way she wants things done.

WIFE: That is *not* true — I wish you showed a little more initiative and did decide at least something every once in a while.

HUSBAND (interrupting): You'd never let me do this!

WIFE: I'd gladly let you — only if I do, nothing ever happens, and then I have to do everything at the last moment.

HUSBAND (to therapist): Can you see? Things can't be taken care of if and when they come up — they have to be planned and organized a week ahead.

WIFE (angrily): Give me *one* example in the last few years when you did do something.

HUSBAND: I guess I can't — because it is better for everybody, including the children, if I let you have your own way. I found this out very early in our marriage.

WIFE: You have never behaved differently, right from the start you didn't — you have always left everything up to me.

HUSBAND: For heaven's sake, now listen to this (pause, then to therapist) — I guess what she is talking about now is that I would always ask her what *she* wanted — like "where would you like to go tonight?" or "what would you like to do over the weekend?" and instead of seeing that I wanted to be nice to her, she would get mad at me ...

WIFE (to therapist): Yeah, what he still doesn't understand is that if you get this "anything-you-want-dear-is-all-right-with-me" stuff, month after month, you begin to feel that nothing you want matters to him.

In both of these examples, the couple is following a rule in which the wife initiates everything and the husband responds to her initiative by agreeing. The pattern leaves both wives uncertain about how their husbands really feel about anything. Neither wife is happy with the arrangement. It could be argued that they have more power than they want. They do not want to decide on everything. They want their husbands to clarify what they really think, and to take charge of something. The husband in example 2 states the typical assumption of husbands caught in this pattern. He assumes that if he does initiate something, his wife will disapprove of whatever it is. To avoid her disapproval, he just turns all decisions over to her. He then becomes invisible.

The husband's spontaneity is not the only thing that these types of patterns regulate. They also regulate the partner's emotional proximity. When and under what circumstances they display affection are regulated by this pattern. They are affectionate when the wife initiates affection, and only then.

We now have observed some of the factors involved in making men disappear: a wife who demands something and becomes upset if her husband disagrees, and a husband who patronizes his wife to avoid her becoming upset. If this sequence becomes a chronic pattern, then the husband never spontaneously initiates behaviors that would clarify his position on a given issue, and the wife is left uncertain as to how he feels about that issue.

The "Be Spontaneous" Paradox

As stated earlier, if a wife becomes uncertain about some important issue, there will be tension between the partners until that uncertainty is clarified and only spontaneous initiatives by the husband will make his position clear. However, this is what the pattern the couple is in will not allow. If the wife becomes uncertain about an important issue and realizes that her husband is not behaving in a way that clarifies his position, she may attempt to get him to explain how he really feels. If she stays within her role, she may take the initiative to get her husband to respond spontaneously. But this is a paradox. Spontaneous behavior cannot be a response to someone else's initiative. The husband cannot be spontaneous in response to a request, either direct or indirect, to be so. The couple is caught in a paradox.

The "be spontaneous" paradox creates a dilemma for both husbands and wives, and for mothers and fathers. In the arrangement in which the woman initiates and the man responds, the man is in a one-down position as the one who never initiates anything. There are two problems: First, to equalize the relationship, the husband's status must be elevated. However, in any relationship with a power imbalance, the more powerful spouse is not in a position to elevate the status of the one-down spouse. The very act of attempting to elevate a one-down partner puts the partner attempting to help in the one-up position. Power cannot be equalized by the more powerful party's magnanimously giving up his or her power. Again, the act of doing this defines the person as more powerful. To equalize the relationship, the one-down party must elevate himself or herself by being assertive and taking some initiative. Second, when the wife is uncertain about some issue because the husband is sending double messages, action initiated by the husband is what is needed for him to make his position clear.

Three Contracts That Make Men Disappear

There are three common methods that couples use in an attempt to solve this problem that can make the situation worse. Each method results in a particular pattern and leads to the way in which a couple may present the problem to professionals.

1. Demand spontaneous behavior.

One problematic pattern is: The wife initiates everything and the husband responds. The wife initiates sex. The wife initiates what will be done with free time. The wife initiates how money will be spent. The wife may say, "Let's go out to dinner." The husband then makes reservations. The wife may decide that a new sofa is needed, and the husband then helps to purchase it. The husband never initiates; he only responds. This could be described as a rigidly complementary relationship in which the wife chronically overfunctions by initiating everything and the husband chronically underfunctions by only responding.

If a wife notices that her husband is not initiating anything, she may request that he do so. She may come to realize that he never initiates affection. Since he never initiates affection, the wife may begin to question whether he really loves her. Or if he never initiates sex, she may begin to wonder whether he still finds her desirable. In an attempt to solve this problem, she may then ask that he initiate affection. This, of course, is not the solution. What typically occurs if the wife requests affection is that the husband then dutifully offers it, and the wife is not satisfied because she had to ask for it.

2. Arrange for spontaneous behavior.

If a wife realizes that she cannot solve a problem by requesting spontaneous behavior, she can attempt to arrange for it by behaving in such a way that requires a response. A problem can be developed to which the husband will have to respond. One could become seriously depressed, or very irresponsible, or manifest serious physiological symptoms, hoping that the noninitiator will then respond "spontaneously" and offer some assistance. Further problems arise if the noninitiator does not respond. Then the initiator must escalate the original problem to try to get a response. A pattern of escalating symmetry may develop. The wife will become more and more depressed or behave in a more and more extreme manner until the husband finally responds. Then, if she deescalates, he returns to his noninitiating posture. He only initiates when she becomes extreme. Again, the partners' emotional proximity is regulated by this pattern. When she exhibits extreme behavior, he becomes attentive, and perhaps even nurturing. When she settles down and begins to get back to normal, he withdraws.

This pattern seems to occur when the husband is struggling with some problem of his own. The wife may then distract him from his difficulty by developing her own problem. A rule develops where by the wife must have a symptom and the husband must help her with her symptom. The husband can then pull himself together and focus on helping his wife.

One crucial aspect of this contract is its implicit nature. The partners do not discuss or acknowledge the husband's struggles. Perhaps he has lost a job, or is in a mid-life crisis, or is grappling with some other important aspect of his life. For whatever reason, he may be vulnerable and insecure. But the husband's having a problem does not in itself set the stage for a quid pro quo in which the wife exhibits a symptom. There also has to be a rule that the husband cannot admit aloud to having a problem, or to being vulnerable, a rule that is not uncommon among men in our society.

If the husband is struggling with a problem, but must deny having a problem, then the wife's dilemma is how to help a man who does not admit he is in trouble. One way to approach the problem is for the wife to help from a one-down position. She may develop a problem of her own, one more serious than the husband's, thus allowing him to be in the position of helping her. He can be distracted from what is bothering him by having to help his wife, and he can raise his self-esteem by assuming the helping role. Although this may aid the husband, it is an unfortunate contract for the wife, who is sacrificing herself in the interest of helping her husband. In such cases, the wife can end up exhibiting serious symptoms and can seek therapy for herself.

3. Get a third person involved.

Partners stuck in a rigidly complementary relationship, or in one that leads to escalating symmetry, are in an unstable relationship and almost always triangulate around a third person to stabilize the situation. The third person could be a lover. When one cannot negotiate with one's spouse, one response is to find someone else. If one of the spouses has psychosomatic or psychological symptoms, the third person might be a professional, such as a medical doctor or a therapist. Sometimes the third person is an in-law or a close friend.

Perhaps the most common third person is one of the children. When the husband has disappeared, the result often is an arrangement in which the mother becomes very involved with one of the children and the father is not so involved. This arrangement can lead to serious problems if the child develops some difficulty. Because the pattern is for the mother to be involved with the child, the father stays uninvolved, even if the child's problem worsens. His silence can then call into question his position regarding the child's behavior. The child, the mother, or both may begin to see the father's inaction as his tolerating the child's behavior or as the father's passively siding with the child against the mother. The child's behavior will then escalate until the father is forced to take a stand. Then the child may settle down and the whole process starts over. The father only takes a position when confronted with extreme behavior on the part of the child. These types of contracts culminate with a child's being presented to therapy as having a problem.

Quid Pro Quo and the Family Life Cycle

A couple appeared on a pop psychology show as an example of how to achieve perfect equality. Before getting married, the couple had set down in detail what each would be responsible for. They worked out who would do what chore, how money would be allocated, what day of the week would be devoted to fun, and who would decide what they would do on those fun days. All of this was negotiated verbally to each one's complete satisfaction. As I watched this couple, I asked myself, "What happens when they have a baby?"

Whatever quid pro quo, satisfactory or not, a given couple has worked out, it has been tailored to fit the life-cycle stage the partners are in. A completely new contract is required when a new stage begins. If partners insist on rigidly adhering to their earlier contract, they can be in trouble when the life cycle requires a change. The idea, first proposed by Haley (1973), is that when a rigid pattern clashes with an irresistible pressure to change, the result often is someone's developing a symptom.

In looking closely at what changes the life cycle requires, we see changes in such things as membership in a family and a household, as well as in status, role, and emotional proximity among intimates. Couples that rigidly obey a particular rule in their relationship may encounter serious difficulty when facing changes of the magnitude that life-cycle shifts demand. Changing who is close to whom, who is distant from whom, and who has power and influence over whom in a family means changing the fundamental aspects of relationships. Not coincidentally, these are the same interpersonal things that symptoms typically regulate.

Changing any of these characteristics of a family requires renegotiations of countless issues, and poses new dilemmas that must be confronted. For example; suppose partners work out a relationship of living separate and independent lives. Both are career minded. Then they have a baby. It is difficult to live separate lives focusing on both careers when they have an infant to whom they must attend. A new contract is required. Another common dilemma in today's culture is how to place equal emphasis on two careers. As each spouse moves up the career ladder, eventually one will be offered an opportunity that cannot be had without the other's sacrificing his or her career. Suppose the wife is offered a promotion but it means moving to another city, which would inhibit the husband's career opportunities. No matter what they decide, their decision inevitably must favor one career over the other. They will have to give up the rule that both careers are to be equally emphasized.

Any of the new dilemmas posed by a life-cycle shift can cause a breakdown in negotiations, and a man who withdraws from those negotiations is a man who becomes invisible.

A life-cycle change can also pose a baffling dilemma that puts a man in the middle between two people and requires him to clarify where he stands on something. For example, after having a new baby, the husband's mother, who previously was not very involved with the couple, now becomes very involved in ways that upset his wife. This is a man caught between two women, and he must make a choice. Some men have difficulty with this. It is not the choice he makes that renders him invisible, it is his uncertainty about what to do that results in his not clarifying how involved he thinks his mother should be. The problem arises from his not clarifying his position. This same problem of a husband, or father, not clarifying his position on something is common in several life-cycle shifts, for example, when a daughter becomes a young woman. The daughter may have been a paternal favorite, and she may be blossoming at a time when her mother feels she herself is fading. The situation can become very volatile, depending on how the man deals with it. If he is invisible, and not making it clear that his wife is the female he prefers, the result probably will be jealousy on the part of both.

Life-cycle changes can also result in a man's being caught between his wife and his boss. As he advances in his career, his profession may make increasing demands on his time that affect his family, and at some point, he will have to take a stand, either with his boss or with his wife. Again, not making a decision can result in serious problems.

These various dilemmas can create a man who is lost, uncertain about what to do, and in trouble. But he is often not the one who is the focus of any professionals involved. The mother of the blossoming daughter is typically the parent who takes the girl in for help, and this is usually a hostile and argumentative dyad. Professionals can easily be persuaded to see just the mother and the daughter together, or the daughter alone, and miss the fact that it is the father's uncertainty about how to intervene that is fueling the hostilities.

What Can Women Do?

When a woman is paired up with an invisible man, what can she do? She may not want to do anything. Some women are satisfied with this arrangement. But if she wants a man to change, how does one change an invisible man? The standard approaches seem to be to nag or provoke. Nagging, however, keeps the woman in the one-up position. If a man responds to nagging, he is implicitly agreeing that he will obey. This may be satisfying initially, but if the woman wants a man with a backbone, then he cannot be one who can be bossed.

Provoking also seems to have some popularity. When faced with a limp noodle, one can try to pick an argument with him. Maybe this might provoke a strong response. The problem here is that, even if it works, the only time the husband actually gets out of his recliner and puts away his remote control is when he and his wife are fighting. Ultimately, this does not satisfy either partner. If the standard approaches are not workable, what else can be tried? There are a number of possibilities.

The woman can try to renegotiate a new contract. She can try to change an implicit contract by negotiating explicitly. She can ask the man what he wants in exchange for his being more involved in the marriage or with the children. The rules of negotiation are that both parties must state their cases, no one is allowed to agree to something he or she is not enthusiastic about, and a successful negotiation ends with both parties feeling as though they won. If one feels like a loser, then a successful settlement has not been reached.

If direct negotiation fails, or if the man refuses to negotiate, the woman can try to change her end of the contract. If her end of the current arrangement is to wash his clothes and iron his shirts, she can go on strike. If her end of the deal is to be assertive and take charge all of the time, she can become inactive. If she is usually the responsible one, she might try being irresponsible. Whatever she is doing on her end, she can begin to do the opposite. Hopefully this will bring the man to the bargaining table, and the woman can then go back to attempting to negotiate.

If the woman has tried to negotiate and that has failed, and changing her end of the contract has also failed, she can attempt to motivate the man by leaving, or threatening to leave. It is hard to leave an invisible man, however. This is not a man who is violent or drinks too much. In all likelihood, this is a man who is mild-mannered, and is not addicted to any of the typical vices. When a man is invisible, it is not obvious what he is doing that is so bad. The main problem might be that he is boring. A woman who wants to leave such a man, is not likely to be supported by her family, or her children. How does she explain the problem? "I'm leaving him because he does everything I ask!" This explanation is not going to be accepted by anyone.

She can try to help him from a one-down position. She can develop a problem in an attempt to organize him. But this creates the unfortunate scenario described earlier. It may raise his self-esteem, or distract him from his problems, but it creates a need for the wife to have a problem.

She can go for help. This also ends up being risky. If she goes into therapy, the therapist might not recognize that she has an invisible man on her hands. The therapist might not see him. Instead, the therapist might send the woman to the doctor for medication, solidifying the arrangement of her being the patient and the man remaining invisible.

On the other hand, if the woman is married and a therapist does recognize that she has a problem husband, the therapist might advise the woman to leave him. This is a problem if what the woman wants is a changed husband, not a divorce.

If the therapist passes the first two tests, recognizing that the husband has a problem and that the woman wants him changed, not gone, the therapist must still pass a third trial. The therapist must understand that the husband must be treated with kid gloves. If the rule is not to talk about his insecurities, then dragging him in to therapy to help him have insight into his problems may end up scaring him off, and negate all her efforts.

Clearly, when a therapist is introduced, the problem is not a simple one. It is a human inclination to want to side with the underdog. A therapist confronted with a couple where either the husband or the wife is one down may be tempted to side with the spouse whose status needs to be raised. With the support of a therapist, the one-down spouse may be able to deal with the partner as an equal, but this is not a solution. In this arrangement, the one-down spouse is only equal when in coalition with a therapist. To truly equalize the relationship, the one-down spouse must initiate something to raise his or her own status. The therapist's task in this situation is to inspire the one-down spouse to take some action that simultaneously raises his or her status and clears up any uncertainty about where he or she stands on important issues. To make an invisible man visible, the therapist must get him to take action, not just talk. What is said in a therapist's office may not be important if it is not followed up with action in real life. Clearly, if therapy is sought by a couple in these unfortunate circumstances, special therapeutic procedures are required. These procedures will be our next topic.

2

Strategies for Engaging and Changing Men

The approach used with the men in this book can be described as Strategic Therapy (Haley, 1973) or as Directive Therapy (Haley, 1996). This approach essentially draws on the intervention techniques of Milton Erickson (Haley, 1967, 1973; Madanes, 1981, 1984, 1990) organized around and guided by the family life cycle (Haley, 1973), and an understanding of family structure (Haley, 1976; Minuchin, 1974; Minuchin & Fishman, 1981). Although the approach has been described at length elsewhere, concepts will be emphasized here that are relevant to working with invisible men specifically.

Assume People Are Trying to Help and Protect Each Other

Haley has proposed that the best theory of motivation for a therapist is the theory that clients are motivated to help someone (Haley, 1996). It is assumed in this approach that a client's symptoms are partly a result of a misguided attempt to be helpful. Although this assumption may not be true in all cases, Haley argues that it is the best stance for a therapist. It makes the client more human and thus an easier subject for the therapist's compassion.

In this way of thinking, for example, a wife who stays home out of fear that she might have a panic attack is attempting to help her insecure husband. This assumption has major implications for creating an invisible man, and for how to work with him. Although, on one hand, the wife's symptom may help her husband pull himself together, and may elevate him to the status of her helper, it also distracts the attention from him and puts it on her. Her protectiveness of him makes him invisible to helpers.

Often the professionals who are consulted make the wife the focus of interventions, and completely miss the fact that she is sacrificing herself to help her husband. The idea that she is helping him also implies that she is protective of him. If asked directly by professionals whether her husband is part of the problem, she is likely to say that he is not, wanting to avoid the possibility of his being confronted by a benevolent helper.

The assumption that a married woman suffering from some symptom is attempting to help her husband leads to a therapy that includes the husband. It also guides the therapist on how to treat the husband. If the wife is protective of him, he will have to be treated with respect and care.

Assuming that a client is motivated to protect someone implies that the client's symptom has an interpersonal function. The symptom has a goal within the client's social milieu. The goal could be to bring two people closer together, or to push two people further apart. It could be to keep someone from leaving or to get rid of someone. Or it could be that the goal of the symptom is to inspire someone to take action to compose himself or herself. Typically, when a wife comes to therapy displaying serious symptoms, we assume that her goal is one of these possibilities.

Think of Families as the Ultimate Self-Help Group

If a woman is having panic attacks as a way to help her husband and she does not want him to become the object of any attention that might be negative, then the question becomes how to organize the therapy. If the wife is helping her husband by having a problem, then it would seem obvious that the simplest way to help the wife with her problem would be to help the husband with his. But if the wife does not want the husband to be implicated in any way, then how can he be helped without identifying him as having a problem?

In the approach offered here, the family is thought of as the ultimate self-help group (Madanes, 1991), and organized to help clients overcome their problems. This is done not only to break patterns in the family that might be perpetuating the problem, but also because we believe that it is simply the most expedient way to solve a problem. The more individuals one can organize to accomplish a given goal, the more likely it is that the goal will be attained.

If the husband is going to be included in therapy, therapists need a philosophy that allows them to approach the husband in a way that will enlist his cooperation and avoid making him defensive. Thinking of the husband as a potential helper, as opposed to being the cause of the problem, is what is proposed here.

This technique has major implications for finding a way to engage men in therapy. The approach presented in this book is to accept the wife's definition of the problem, and to invite the husband in as a helper to the therapist. He can be approached as the person who knows his wife best and is in the best position to help her. If a wife is concerned about whether or not her husband will participate in therapy, it is assumed that approaching him in this way will please her. If the husband has problems about which the wife is concerned, or if the husband needs to change the way he is treating his wife, these changes can be asked for within the framework of what the husband will have to do differently in order to help his wife. The husband can be approached respectfully, but still be asked to change.

The Therapeutic Relationship

Do Not Offer Help Unless Help Is Requested

A woman comes home after a hard day at the office. She begins to recount her day to her husband, listing the various events that bothered her. After about five minutes, the husband starts offering her advice on how to improve her work situation. The wife becomes annoyed with her husband, saying that she does not want his help to fix the problem, she just wanted to unwind. The wife was not asking for help in changing anything. The husband was offering advice without being invited to do so. Trouble can occur in any relationship if one party offers advice without having been asked. Therapists would be wise to remember this.

The first step in helping a man is to get him to request it. Not only must a man ask for help, but what he seeks help with must be a solvable problem. Sometimes this requires negotiation. Studies support the ideas that focusing on specific problems and negotiating with men on what is in it for them are two important factors in engaging them in therapy (Heubeck, 1986; Hecker, 1991).

A man in his 40s came to therapy because he said his wife insisted that he get help. They had been married for 19 years and had two teenage children. Since the birth of the children, he and his wife had an arrangement in place whereby he worked and provided for the family while she stayed at home and raised the children. Now that the children were in their late teens, the wife decided, to the her husband's consternation, that she was going to go back to school and get a degree in computer programming. The husband was suddenly on his own to make himself dinner every night and to do his own laundry. What was even more upsetting to him was his wife's desire to attend computer conferences. That required her to be away for entire weekends. She had never done anything like this before during their marriage. The man wanted help in persuading his wife to drop out of school and to go back to taking care of him. This obviously was not a therapeutic goal to which a therapist could agree.

The therapist asked the man if he was lonely and missed his wife. He admitted that he did, explaining that they had grown apart and that their relationship had become very distant. He had hoped that when the children were older he could reconnect with her, but then she went back to school. "So the real problem is that you want to be closer to your wife?," the therapist asked. "Right," answered the man. "Does she really have to sacrifice her school to get closer to you?" the therapist asked. "Not really," the man replied. The therapist asked the man if he would be interested in being helped to get closer to his wife, even if that meant her staying in school. The man said that he would and admitted that his constant moping and complaining about her absence was probably just turning her off. The therapist then asked if the man would be willing to try some new things with his wife to see whether she might respond to him more positively. The man was very interested, as he was essentially asking for advice on how to win his wife back. A solvable problem was negotiated, with the man making a clear request for help with that problem. The therapist was now in a position to give advice.

Make Therapy Personal

Somehow a notion has arisen that Strategic therapists are more concerned about fancy therapy strategies than about the therapeutic relationship with the client. In Strategic Therapy, an approach that relies heavily on the client's completing tasks assigned by the therapist, the therapeutic relationship is its most important aspect. Few men or women are going to follow the advice of a therapist whom they do not trust, or whom they feel does not understand them.

It is our assumption that men respond positively when they feel that the therapist is taking a personal interest in them as individuals. This means that to be successful with the most dire cases, the therapist must become intensely and personally involved, which usually requires the therapist to do something that demonstrates to the client that he or she is really interested in helping. It might mean making a home visit, tracking down relatives to engage in the therapy, purchasing something especially for the client that may help the client overcome a problem, or visiting a client in a hospital. What is important is that the therapist do something that shows the client that the client is not just the therapist's 27th appointment that week.

Milton Erickson was a master of this approach. He met clients at restaurants to help them over anxiety, he went to their homes to play jacks with them or race bicycles against them; he made clear efforts to demonstrate a personal interest in his clients.

Mary had been in a psychiatric hospital for over 10 years. She was diagnosed as schizophrenic and sat in a corner all day, every day, not communicating with anyone. A young intern, Rhonda Burnaugh, took an interest in Mary and was determined to connect with her. She had read Mary's history and knew that Mary had been admitted to the hospital after setting herself on fire. Mary recovered from her burns, but had not communicated with anyone and had not done so during her entire stay in the hospital. Every day for two weeks, Rhonda would sit next to Mary and talk to her. But Mary would just ignore her visits and sometimes seem irritated.

Finally, one day Rhonda insisted that some fresh air would be good for Mary and that they should go for a walk. At first, Mary ignored the idea, but Rhonda stood over her and continued to insist that a walk would be good for her. Then, suddenly, Mary spoke. She declared she did not want to go outside and wished to be left alone. To the staff's knowledge, this was the first time anyone in the hospital had heard Mary speak. Rhonda did not give up. Every day, she would sit with Mary and push her to go out for a walk. Finally, Mary agreed to the idea and soon they were taking daily walks and Mary began to talk more.

After many walks, Rhonda asked Mary why she had set herself on fire those many years ago. Mary told an incredible story. At the time, she was a nun and had been having an affair with a priest. When she became pregnant, the priest broke off the affair. To protect the priest, Mary had an abortion and kept their relationship a secret. She was devastated about the whole turn of events. Distraught over the priest's abandoning her and feeling guilty about the abortion, she tried to kill herself by lighting herself on fire. At the time of her suicide attempt, she was the one hospitalized, but there was a man in the background who was a large part of the problem. The man was overlooked because Mary protected him. She was then diagnosed as insane and hospitalized for 10 years.

Rhonda took a personal interest in Mary as a human being, not as a curiosity. Mary responded by trusting Rhonda and telling her story. Once her story was told, her "illness" became more comprehensible. She continued to improve and was eventually released from the hospital, remaining in contact with Rhonda for over 10 years after her release through letters and cards. To Rhonda's knowledge, Mary was never rehospitalized. We assume that all clients have a story that, if told, would make their problems more understandable. But to accomplish this, a therapist first must win the client's trust. As in any therapy approach, in Strategic Therapy this is the first and most important step.

ENGAGING MEN

When a child or a wife has a problem, what difference does it make if the father or husband participates in therapy? This question will be explored in detail in the two chapters dealing with these respective problems.

First, let us consider the problem of how to get a man to participate in therapy. When this question was raised at a conference on brief therapy, many therapists in the audience reported difficulty with accomplishing it. The answer suggested to the therapists was simple. Just call them up and invite them. This seems so ridiculously easy that it hardly seems necessary to point it out. But it has been my experience as a supervisor and trainer of therapists that if a wife or a mother and child come in without the husband or father, many therapists will proceed for several sessions, if not for the entire course of therapy, without inviting the man. If the man then is invited, it is often after several sessions, and so if he does agree to attend, he is coming into a process that is already in progress without any input from him.

It would appear that research confirms the view that starting child therapy without the father has a great bearing on whether or not treatment will be completed for that child. LaBarbera and Lewis (1980) reported that 72% of families continued treatment and followed through with recommendations when the father attended the first therapy session. In contrast, only 47% did so when the father was not included in the first session. LaFave (1980) reported remarkably similar results, finding that 69% of families remained in treatment if the father attended the first session whereas only 44% remained in treatment if he did not.

It has been my experience, both as a therapist and as a supervisor, that if the man is invited to the first session, (or even the second session, if he did not come the first time), he will come a vast majority of the time. Assuming that the therapist is not blaming them for the problem, but is inviting them to provide input and to help solve a problem, few men will refuse a therapist's invitation. Research seems to back up this view.

Heubeck (1986) and Hecker (1991) offer tips for engaging fathers in therapy that are a compilation of several studies (L'Abate, 1975; Stanton & Todd, 1982) and also can be directly applied to engaging husbands of symptomatic wives. These tips include:

- Personally invite the father or husband to the initial session and offer a rationale for why he is needed: "So I can get your point of view and understand the full picture."
- Invite the father or husband to express his wishes for the therapy: "What would you like to see happen about your child's (wife's) therapy?"
- Acknowledge that the man's goals for treatment may be different from those of other family members.
- Keep the focus on the presenting problem as proof of the family's need for his participation, emphasizing his responsibility to contribute and the fact that change may depend on his participation.
- Be willing to work around the father's or husband's work schedule. Offer choices.

On rare occasions, it might be necessary to make a special effort to visit the man on his turf. Dale McClure is a home-based therapist who works with rural families who have a child at risk of being placed in foster care. To avoid doing so, Children's Services assigns Dale to the case to try to resolve whatever family issue is placing the child at risk. These families typically do not seek help on their own and the men in the families in particular probably would not venture within a hundred miles of a mental health center if they could avoid it. Nevertheless, Dale manages to engage these men in therapy, and even to get them to change how they are conducting themselves. He does this by visiting them on their turf, making a special effort to join with them, and convincing them that they can play an important part in solving the problem at hand. One father with whom he worked was a construction worker who had refused to see anyone from Children's Services. Dale spent an afternoon with him while they installed insulation. The man lived with his wife, a teenage stepdaughter, and his wife's mother, and admitted that he felt that he had no status in the home. Because Dale sought him out at his work, where he had status and took pride in what he did, the man was initially seen where he was at his best. He ended up telling his life story to Dale, who was then in a position to suggest to the man that he do some things differently.

Another man who had been refusing to participate was a truck driver and Dale met him at a truck stop. Dale achieved the same results as he did with the construction worker. One reason he was able to accomplish this was that he was committed to get them involved. Obviously not all therapists can join a man on his job for an afternoon, but if Dale can engage men who are not requesting help and who would be very resistant to therapy, the rest of us ought to be able to get many of the men from the families with which we work to come to sessions.

Once the men are engaged in therapy and can agree on an issue that they themselves think needs to change, then what? How does one help a man to change? He can be coached, he can be mentored, or he can be provoked. One can get under his skin, or one can compete with him. He can be challenged, his ego can be stroked, he can be nurtured, or he can be reasoned with. Can a woman therapist do these types of things as effectively as a man can? Many probably can do some of these things more effectively than many men therapists and vice versa. I know a young female therapist who was able to persuade a husband with whom she was working to make major changes in the way he treated his wife. She offered him tips from a woman's point of view on how women like to be treated. The husband obviously viewed the young therapist as someone who could offer some very good pointers on such matters, and so he allowed her to become his coach. The therapist took advantage of her personal characteristics to find a way to connect with this man and to offer him advice.

Pay Attention to Details

A simple way to demonstrate one's personal interest is to *devise a unique plan for each case*. Once the therapist understands a man's situation, he or she can offer a strategy tailored to help that particular man. This approach entails a greater responsibility on the part of the therapist and requires that the therapist have a detailed understanding of the man's dilemma. When trying to understand the rituals associated with symptoms, one goal is for the therapist to be able to visualize exactly what is happening. Pursuing the client for such details is one way for a therapist to demonstrate intense interest in the client's problem and to help the therapist to devise a unique strategy for each case. Again, Milton Erickson was a pioneer in this. One of Erickson's clients was a woman with a severe case of compulsive washing (Haley, 1973). She would wash herself for as many as 20 hours a day. In his initial session with her, Erickson asked, "When you get into the shower to scrub yourself for hours, do you start at the top of your head, or the soles of your feet, or in the middle? Do you wash from the neck down, or do you start with your feet and wash up?" When asked why he posed these questions, Erickson said, "So she would know I was really interested."

Another advantage of pursuing details is that often understanding the details of the client's rituals will lead to an idea about what to do. If a therapist can visualize exactly what is happening when the symptom occurs, or if the family can enact it in the therapist's office, it is easier to understand what to do. It is when a therapist is in tune with the client that an idea about how to intervene will come to mind.

Give Advice

One way in which a therapist can help a man change is to direct him to behave differently. Giving directives is a hallmark of Strategic Therapy and is typically thought of as the approach's major intervention technique. But giving directives is not just aimed at facilitating change. Giving directives defines the relationship between therapist and client. When directives are given, therapy becomes more personal. Clients have to decide whether or not they are going to follow the advice. The therapist drives home wondering if the advice offered to the client will be helpful, whether the client will follow through on the task, and what will happen if he or she does. Haley (1992) gives the example of the Zen master and the student. The Zen master gives the student the task of sweeping the floor or setting up a tea party. The point of the instruction is not to teach about tea parties. Giving the directives connects the two individuals and defines their relationship. In therapy, as in Zen, the advice given is not the point. The giving of the advice defines the process and the relationship.

When giving advice to a man (or to any client), it is important to understand that it is not the directive itself that will solve the problem. The curative aspect of giving directives comes from how the client responds to being told what to do by another human being. The relationship between therapist and client is what gives directives their power. I once worked with a man who was facing retirement and was lost about what he was going to do. His wife was concerned about him and arranged for an appointment. I suggested, rather emphatically, that he become a Christian missionary. He was adamantly opposed to this idea. I insisted. He found himself in the ridiculous position of having a younger man, who was not even close to retiring, giving him advice on what to do in his retirement. My directing him inspired him to think more deeply and to decide what he wanted to do after he retired. He then came in to inform me how ludicrous my idea was, and that he had come up with his own plan. The specific advice I gave was irrelevant. What helped was how the man responded to being told what to do by a younger man.

One issue concerns the question of whether therapy is collaborative if the therapist gives advice. Does the act of giving advice put the therapist in a one-up position, and thus interfere with therapy as a collaborative process? When considering verbal communication, intonation, and body movements, Birdwhistell (1970) estimated that two individuals in communication exchange 100,000 bits of information per minute. It is our assumption that when a therapist is really interested in, and engaged with, a client, and an idea suddenly comes to mind about what to do, the source of that inspiration was the rapport between therapist and client. The creativity comes in part from the client, and when a therapist is in rapport with the client, he or she is in touch with the client's creativity. In this sense, if the proper relationship exists between client and therapist, it is impossible for the therapy not to be collaborative. The therapist's mind is stimulated by the interchange with the client and the advice given, therefore, is partly a product of the client's contribution to the process. Establishing a collaborative process between therapist and client is not a function of whether or not the therapist takes an "expert" posture with the client or gives directives. Collaboration is a function of the therapeutic relationship. If the therapist is interested and is paying attention, the chances are that the process is collaborative.

The Unchangeable Pattern Meets the Irresistible Force

In Strategic Therapy, the unit of analysis involves at least three persons. To understand a particular man's dilemma, it helps to think in threes. As has been noted elsewhere, with three individuals, there is the possibility of coalitions between two of them against the third (Haley, 1967). More fundamentally, with three individuals, an organization with a hierarchy can develop. To be functional, organizations must follow certain rules. One rule that Haley (1996) points out is that a viable organization requires three levels. The third level is needed in order to define the other two. For example, a manager has no authority over a staff unless upper management informs the staff that the manager is in charge. Or, with a family, one parent can have no authority over the children unless the other parent tells the children they have to listen. When a therapist is introduced into the picture, it is important that the therapist understand how to enter the family as an organization to produce the change the family seeks. Understanding the family as an organization (Minuchin, 1974; Minuchin & Fishman, 1981) provides the therapist with a map of how to intervene. When considering how to influence an organization, one must be concerned about the subsystems of that organization, the power structure, the coalitions, and the boundaries, and consider how introducing oneself into that system will shift it in one way or another.

Thinking of an invisible man as following a contract in a marriage defines the problem as dyadic. The couple becomes the unit, and a couple does not constitute an organization with a hierarchy. But a couple that cannot negotiate is an unstable unit. Even if each partner has the best intentions to have an equal marriage and is willing to negotiate in good faith, sooner or later, partners will likely be faced with an issue that they as a couple cannot resolve and continue to remain equals.

For example, one way to resolve an issue is for one of the partners to develop a symptom. If the couple cannot agree on how much work the husband should do around the house, the husband can develop a bad back. His bad back then becomes the basis for deciding what he can and cannot do around the house. The problem is that the wife may then want the husband to see a doctor about his bad back. A third person thus is brought in, presumably to render an opinion on what the husband can and cannot do because of his back. When a problem develops, the dyad quickly becomes a triad. With an unstable couple, the third person could be an in-law, a friend, a therapist, or a child.

When a therapist enters the picture, if there is no third person apparent, then the therapist should consider himself or herself the third person. The couple comes to therapy wanting the therapist to help them make a decision about some dilemma. The therapist must then decide how to handle the issue of what coalition, if any, to be in. Will the therapist side with the wife or with the husband? Or try to remain neutral? Whatever the therapist decides, when working with couples, the minimum unit is three: husband, wife, and therapist.

Whoever the third person may be, if the partners are not able to resolve their issues, the third person's involvement can become chronic. Rigid patterns may develop that require all three individuals. And if having a relationship that requires a third party is not bad enough, the situation can really heat up when a life-cycle change is looming, putting pressure on all parties to adapt to a new situation. In this approach, problems are understood as partly resulting from a clash between repeating rigid patterns and the life cycle's requiring a change in those patterns. When the problem involves an invisible man, often the man is ambivalent and uncertain about how to adjust to a life-cycle change that includes himself and two other individuals. The two other individuals could vary among a number of candidates: his wife and daughter, his wife and his boss, his wife and his mother, his wife and ex-wife, his lover and his father, his son and second wife, and so on. If he is uncertain how to react to a new situation involving any two important people in his life, he may become immobilized, and not assert himself to define his position regarding the issue. His inaction makes him invisible and creates an ambivalent situation for everyone involved.

How to Intervene

TAKE SIDES

Minuchin was the first to introduce the term "unbalancing" (Minuchin & Fishman, 1981). The idea is for a therapist purposely to side with one spouse against the other. If partners come to therapy, each wanting the therapist to side with him or her against the other, the therapist is under considerable pressure to do so. It would seem that remaining neutral is what would be best, but thinking from a systemic point of view reveals otherwise. When a client or couple seeks therapy, the introduction of a therapist into the system forces the family to deal with a new relationship: therapist and client. If one goal of therapy is to change relationship patterns among intimates, then a therapist's remaining neutral will mean siding equally with all individuals in the system. If everyone in the system is influenced equally by the therapist, the system will remain the same. To change the system, the therapist must exert unequal influence. The therapist must join with one side of the system against another to get both sides to shift. The introduction of the therapist into the system is being used to bring about a change. Changing a circular process requires a linear intervention. This means that a therapist must take sides to help a couple change. The trick is to take sides in a way that will change a rigid pattern, rather than in a way that will reinforce it.

In the broadest sense, a therapist seeing a spouse individually is unbalancing. Individual therapy is taking sides. Unequal influence is being exerted on the couple. Seeing clients individually, or in subgroups, is not necessarily antitherapeutic; it can potentially be a problem, however, if a therapist decides to see a client individually without considering the impact the therapist's presence will have on the client's social context.

A woman in her mid-30s came alone to see me complaining of panic attacks. She was married and had no children. At the end of the first interview, I asked her to bring her husband to the next appointment. I wanted to include him in her treatment, and to get his help in working with her. The husband came in with her the next time, and he was a mess. He was obviously depressed and lethargic, a very passive man. He was having a crisis in his career, was not sure what to do about it, and was very distant from his wife. He was confused, and therefore hesitant to take action at home or at work.

I explained that I had invited him in to ask his help with his wife, and he answered that he did not think he could be of much use to me. He said he had been in therapy for over two years for depression and could barely take care of his own problems. When he mentioned that he was in therapy, his wife erupted. He had been seeing a woman therapist who was performing a Jungian analysis. He saw her weekly and paid her $90 for each visit. In addition to the weekly fee, he was in debt to her for over $2,000. The wife explained that his therapy was a financial burden and was using up all of their discretionary income. I took this to mean that if the wife wanted to buy a new dress, she could not, because her husband was giving the money to another woman. Not only that, but the other woman was learning all of the husband's deepest, darkest secrets. If the wife were told anything, she would be the second woman told, not the first.

I explained to the man privately that I needed his help, and that if he decided to participate, I would ask him to take a recess from his therapy during the time he was working with me. He thought this over and agreed. For the next three weeks, I attempted several times to reach his therapist, but she would not return my calls.

Finally, I called the couple in and explained to the husband that while I was waiting to hear from his therapist, he needed something that he could do that would help if his wife were to have a panic attack. I said that I thought he might be able to shock her out of having an attack, but he would have to be willing to take strong measures. He agreed. I then told him that the next time his wife began to get anxious, he was to drop his pants and his underwear right down to his ankles. I thought this would help distract his wife from having a panic attack.

He did not drop his pants but he did relay my suggestion to his therapist, who promptly called to tell me what a nut I was. After giving me a lecture, the therapist informed me that the man's wife was very pathological. She had no idea how much damage her individual therapy was doing to her client's marriage. She had not considered how, through her therapy, she was intruding on the marriage. After talking about the case, she agreed to release the man temporarily so that I could work with the couple.

Unbalancing is a very powerful intervention if a therapist considers the client's social context and how introducing an expert into that context will bring about a change. Preferably, the partners are brought in together so the therapist can observe the situation, hear each side out, and then make a decision as to whom to meet with and how to intervene. Haley (1996) refers to this as deciding on the unit for therapy. This decision should be made with the client's social context in mind.

There are at least four major ways in which an invisible man can end up in therapy. The man can come in with his wife, with the marriage presented as the problem. He can come in with his family, with one of the children presented as having a problem. He can come in alone, presenting himself as having a problem. Or, if his wife comes to therapy presenting herself as the patient, the husband can be invited in to help. In this approach, after observing the couple or family together, hearing everyone's view of the situation, and gaining rapport with each individual, unbalancing is used to deal with all of these different ways the man can come in. The therapist hears everyone out and then takes a stand about what should be done. The position the therapist takes with respect to what should be done about the problem puts the therapist in a coalition with someone. A peripheral father can be put in charge of a problem child. A neglectful husband can be put in charge of helping his depressed wife. The therapist can take sides in a dispute between two spouses who are at an impasse. All of the cases in this book involve the technique of unbalancing to change rigid patterns in relationships. The art of working with these dyads involves being unafraid to take sides, and understanding what coalition will promote change and what coalition will inhibit it.

CHANGE RITUALS

In this approach, the goal of the therapy is to resolve the presenting problems of the client. This means focusing on specific symptoms. But when viewed through an interpersonal lens, *symptoms are ritualistic behaviors and include everyone who is intimately involved with the symptom bearer.* Haley (1976) refers to the patterns created by symptomatic rituals as interpersonal sequences. As with all human rituals, symptomatic rituals are laden with multiple meanings for all of the participants. Changing symptomatic rituals, therefore, results in changes on multiple levels. When understood on an interpersonal level, it is clear that an individual's symptom can regulate whom that person is emotionally close to or distant from, and for what reason. The symptom can define who has power, when the person has it, and whom he or she has it over. The more serious the problem, the more the problem regulates the daily lives of those who are intimate with the symptomatic individual. Changing symptomatic rituals not only means changing behavior, it also means changing cognition, interpersonal relationships, experiential meanings — and who knows what else? There is much more at stake than changing simple behaviors.

When a therapist clearly understands what a couple's rituals are, it is not difficult to think of multiple changes the couple might make. For example, every night, when her husband came home, one woman would have a gourmet meal prepared. When the couple sat down together to enjoy their meal, without fail, the husband would pick up his *New York Times* and begin to read, ignoring his wife. Also without fail, the wife would begin to stuff herself as soon as her husband began to read. After stuffing herself, the wife would politely excuse herself from the table and go into the downstairs bathroom and vomit. Throughout this bulimic episode, the husband would continue to read his paper. No words would be spoken by either party. That was the couple's ritual.

When thinking about how the couple could change this ritual, a multitude of possibilities come to mind. The wife could announce, before she went to the bathroom, "Your ignoring me makes me sick. I'm going to the bathroom to vomit!" Or, when the wife began to binge at the table, the husband could put his paper down and say, "Vomiting is bad for your health. Please do not do that." Or when the wife dismissed herself to go vomit, the husband could go into the bathroom with her and supervise the vomiting. Or, the wife could go into the bathroom alone and pretend to vomit. She could go through her whole routine, but when in the bathroom, just flush the toilet without vomiting. The husband would think she had vomited, but she would not have.

Any of these changes would be a change in their ritual. It is doubtful whether any of them could take place without other major changes occurring as well, however. In this particular case, the wife was very upset with her husband for various reasons of which he was well aware. At the same time, she was very protective of him and did not want to voice her displeasure. Her vomiting was a silent way of protesting. The couple's dinner ritual was laden with meaning. It was a way of acting out a quid pro quo that was worked out by the couple for many reasons. Asking for any change in their symptomatic ritual would simultaneously force a change in their quid pro quo, and in all of the issues that went into creating that quid pro quo.

Listen Metaphorically/Intervene Literally

A 14-year-old girl was brought into therapy by both of her parents. The girl was convinced she was possessed by spirits and was behaving bizarrely. She was not functioning at school, and at home, isolated herself in her room, fearing it was not safe to venture out. In the first session, the girl was extremely upset and cried the entire time. A reasonable interview was barely possible. The mother was a very religious woman and believed the girl was actually possessed. The father was an engineer and thought his wife's beliefs were absurd. The mother was very anxious about the girl's distress. The father was concerned about his daughter, but annoyed by his wife. The mother was deeply involved with her daughter, whereas the father was very distant from both of them. It seemed obvious that the mother and daughter were a metaphor for each other. They both believed in spirit possession and were both being neglected by the man in the home. At one point in the interview, the father explained that "she" was very upset by the idea that spirits were in the house. The father did not specify to which "she" he was referring and since both the mother and daughter believed in spirit possession, he could have been referring to either.

In this approach, it is recommended that therapists listen metaphorically, but intervene literally. This means that when metaphors are apparent, such as in this example, the therapist should take note of it, but not comment on it. In the above case, for instance, if the father had been comfortable with specifying to whom he was referring, he would have done so. If a therapist tried to pin him down by getting him to specify, or commented aloud that the father was speaking in metaphor, he might regret that he had made the statement and stop communicating metaphorically. The therapist would be stifling communication (Haley, 1996).

Not commenting, however, does not mean that the therapist should ignore the information. In this case, the father was put in charge of helping his daughter with regard to her spirit possession. He was moved from a peripheral position with respect to the problem to a central one. He was told that regardless of his personal beliefs about spirit possession, his daughter actually believed she was possessed, and, therefore, if he were going to help her, he would have to take her belief seriously. This meant he would have to learn about spirit possession. Since his wife was an expert on spirit possession, he would have to ask her to teach him about it. The therapist noted the metaphor, but intervened literally. The father was asked to change how he was interacting with both his wife and his daughter. The man took the task on wholeheartedly. His daughter improved, and so did his marriage.

One advantage of intervening literally is that literal interventions can break up the most severe pathology. A client can present severe psychological symptoms and a therapist can intervene as if the symptoms were literally true. A classic Erickson example involved one of his patients who believed himself to be Jesus Christ (Haley, 1983). He was hospitalized and wandered around all day performing "miracles," but not doing anything that might get him out of the hospital. Erickson approached him and said, "I understand that you are a carpenter." The man had to agree. Erickson then put the man to work doing carpentry. The patient either had to drop his delusion, which would be improvement, or do productive work, which would also be improvement.

John, a 42-year-old man, was driving on the highway one night on a trip to visit his parents. On the car radio, he began to hear Jesus speaking to him. Jesus told him that he would be protected and that he could drive as fast as he wished. John then accelerated to 90 miles an hour. Within seconds, he had slammed into the back of a semi-tractor-trailer truck that was traveling much slower. The car rolled into the ditch, but miraculously, John was uninjured.

Jesus continued to communicate with John and told him that he could walk on the highway opposite the direction of traffic and he would be protected. John then proceeded to walk down the highway at night, opposing traffic. A car sideswiped his arm and injured him severely. John ended up in the hospital.

Rhonda Burnaugh was assigned the case and consulted with the author about making a hospital visit. The problem was that John was only communicating in psychotic babble. No one knew anything about why he did what he did, or how to help him. It was decided that in an attempt to get John to communicate normally, Rhonda would take a radio along when she visited him in the hospital.

The next day, when she entered John's hospital room, she introduced herself as the therapist who would be working with him when he was released from the hospital. After making small talk, she asked him why he had driven so recklessly that night. John mumbled something about Jesus. Rhonda then showed him her radio, saying that she understood that Jesus was communicating with John via his car radio. Rhonda explained that she too wished to communicate with Jesus, and asked John to help her find the station that Jesus was on. She had searched all the channels and could not find him. Was he on AM or FM?

John began to giggle. He put his hand over his mouth and laughed aloud. He then got up and paced around the room, looking over at Rhonda and continuing to laugh. He then became serious and told her what was happening. John explained that he was gay, and had been living with his lover for the past 10 years, but concealed the fact from his parents, telling them that they were roommates. Although John's partner was openly gay, John was reluctant to admit the true situation to his family. Invisibility is not limited to men in heterosexual relationships. Finally, after much agonizing, John decided to assert himself. He would drive to his parents' house and tell them the truth. On his way to his parents, Jesus had intervened; rather than tell his parents the truth, John had attempted suicide.

Intervening literally helped John communicate sensibly. Once he told his story, he expressed regret at not having carried out his plan to tell his secret to his parents. Rhonda and John then planned a strategy whereby John, with Rhonda's help, could inform his parents of his sexual orientation.

Push for Normal Behavior

Although this rule applies in all cases, it primarily concerns clients who are exhibiting the most impaired functioning. It requires courage, but even in the most difficult cases, a therapist must push for, and settle for nothing less than, what would be normal for that person given his or her cultural background, socioeconomic status, and position in the family life cycle. It is assumed here that a normal routine will help return a person to normal ways of thinking and feeling. A classic Haley example is of a woman who became depressed after giving birth to her first child (Haley, 1973). She ended up in the hospital, and when she was released, she found that her husband had moved himself and their child in with his mother, who was now caring for the woman's baby. She was in a completely abnormal situation, and this no doubt was exacerbating her symptoms. Despite her severe depression, Haley pushed the couple to move back into their own apartment at once, creating a situation in which the woman could care for her own baby.

This rule also has implications for when to end therapy. Therapy should end when the client is functioning within the normal range of behavior considering the client's developmental, cultural, and socioeconomic background. An Erickson case can serve as an example of this (Erickson, 1980). A man with numerous psychosomatic symptoms underwent 500 hours of psychoanalysis, but was not helped. He then underwent 500 hours of analysis by a second doctor, and still was not helped. He then was sent to Erickson for "superficial" symptom relief. Erickson found out that the man had been married for 15 years, had three children, and had lived for the entire time next door to his mother. Erickson worked with this man during the early 1950s, and so for that era, it was quite unusual that in their years of marriage, his wife had never cooked breakfast for him. Instead, every morning his mother would come to his house and prepare his breakfast. Not surprisingly, his mother also did many other things to "help" the family.

When the couple first married, they were not permitted to go on a honeymoon. His mother had insisted that her son take two weeks off from work and that they honeymoon in their new home, next to the parents' home. To the bride's horror, the mother showed up the next morning to prepare breakfast. She had decided the menu and the couple had to eat what she prepared. The mother also cooked lunch and the evening meal, in addition to telling them when to go to bed and when to get up. This behavior had continued for the entire 15 years of their marriage. She had strong opinions about what constituted a proper diet, and which liquids were appropriate and which were not. Milk was allowed for children, not for adults. Tea was fine. Soft drinks were out. Alcohol was strictly forbidden. The man was caught between his mother and his wife and was not asserting himself. By not asserting himself, he was not defining what he believed to be an appropriate relationship between his mother and his family. On this issue, he was invisible.

After interviewing the man alone, Erickson invited the wife to join them. She said that the intrusions of her mother-in-law made her very upset, but she had resigned herself to the idea that her husband would never stand up to his mother. After obtaining a commitment from the couple to work together, Erickson proposed a plan whereby they could distance themselves somewhat from the husband's mother. They agreed, and the next morning when the husband's mother came over to cook breakfast, they were ready for her. As soon as she began to bark orders, the wife reached into the cupboard and pulled out a bottle of whiskey. Her mother-in-law was astonished as the wife proceeded to pour a drink. She gave it to her husband, and before the mother could object, the husband drank it down. When the mother protested, the wife responded by pouring her husband a second drink, which he promptly disposed of. The mother was so shocked that she left the house and did not return for three days. These were the first three days that the couple had been together without seeing the husband's mother.

When the mother returned, she began a stern lecture on the evils of alcohol. Her son's response was to reach into his coat pocket, pull out a flask of brown fluid (it was tea, but it passed as whiskey) and begin to drink it. Again, his mother became overwhelmingly disturbed and departed. Erickson then convinced the couple to sell their house and move across town.

At this point, the man's symptoms had abated, but Erickson was not finished. The couple had achieved some distance from the man's mother, but the three were not on speaking terms and this was not normal. Erickson persuaded the couple to ask the mother over for Thanksgiving dinner. The meal began uneventfully, but soon the mother was giving orders as to what everyone should eat and how large their servings should be. Again the family was prepared. Both parents and all three children stood up in unison and left the table. The family then gave the grandmother another chance, inviting her to Christmas dinner. This time, she was very polite, everyone had a nice time, and the case could be closed. Erickson did not terminate this case when the man had overcome his symptoms, but was still in a strained and abnormal relationship with his mother. Instead, Erickson pushed for what, considering their cultural background, would be a more normal way of relating, and stayed with the case until the family had achieved that.

3

Invisible Husbands

TYPICAL PATTERNS

The most common pattern among couples that include an invisible husband is one in which the wife initiates everything and the husband responds to what the wife initiates. The wife initiates sex, the wife initiates spending free time together, the wife instructs the husband when and how to intervene with the children, and so on. When a couple follows this rule, it becomes unclear as to how the husband really feels about anything. If the husband never initiates affection, the wife may begin to doubt how he feels about her. If the husband defers to the wife on all important matters, she will eventually begin to wonder where he stands on anything. By her always taking the initiative, the husband's position on any given issue is never clarified. He is invisible.

A problem that is sometimes associated with couples following this rule is an emotional or sexual withdrawal by the husband. One way in which partners can fall into this pattern is through failed attempts to negotiate. One scenario in which the husband withdraws is this: The wife states her view on an issue, and the husband then presents his. The wife responds by becoming upset, and the husband capitulates. He goes along with her, not because he agrees with her, but because he is intimidated by the intensity of her reaction. He is avoiding her intense reaction. He then becomes resentful and withdraws emotionally or sexually. In extreme cases, he may end up having an affair. The wife may begin to suspect that something is bothering him, but when she inquires, he denies it. To avoid her possibly intense reaction, he says, "Everything is OK, dear."

These couples typically come into therapy at the point at which the *wife* realizes that her husband is not initiating anything. In some cases, she has withdrawn from taking the initiative herself. She may want some sign from him that would clarify how he feels, but this sign will not be forthcoming as long as he continues to follow the rule of deferring to her. On the other hand, he may be confused by her withdrawal from initiating. He may begin to question whether she still loves him. The couple can become stuck in an arrangement in which each is waiting for the other to take the initiative.

Unbalancing Couples

When a therapist intervenes in this type of arrangement, the task at hand is to inspire the one-down spouse to take the initiative spontaneously. One way to accomplish this is to take sides (Minuchin & Fishman, 1981; Haley, 1996). If a therapist attempts to be fair with a couple and to side equally with both spouses, the therapist is simply confirming the arrangement that the couple already is in. To attain a change, the therapist must throw his or her weight in one direction or the other, requiring the couple to react to the therapist's stance by changing their arrangement. The question for the therapist is how to create a coalition that will produce the change desired by the couple, as opposed to reinforcing what the couple already is doing.

Obviously, the act of a therapist's siding with a husband or a wife, each of whom wants the therapist to side with him or her, can easily blow up in the therapist's face if not done properly. To perform this intervention, the therapist must first hear each partner's side of the problem and be in empathic contact with each. Each partner must feel that the therapist understands his or her respective position. With this accomplished, the therapist can take the stand he or she thinks necessary in order for the couple to improve the situation.

The therapist can push one or the other to initiate a change in the name of improving the marriage, or the therapist can take a position that pulls the couple together in relation to the therapist. For example, if one spouse has withdrawn sexually and the other is pushing for sex, the partners can end up in a frustrating situation in which their sexual activity has stopped or greatly diminished. The therapist can take the position that they should not be having sex, but they should emphasize being affectionate. They can touch each other in nonsexual ways to improve being affectionate, but they cannot have sex. Typically, they will rebel against this directive and resume their sexual relationship. In this way of unbalancing, the partners pull together in relation to the therapist.

Another option is for the therapist to side with the wife against the husband, or with the husband against the wife. When the problem is the husband's not initiating anything, whatever coalition the therapist chooses must be aimed at inspiring the husband to take action.

What can cause serious problems is a therapist who takes sides before each spouse has stated his or her respective views. This error can easily occur if one spouse has been seen individually and then the other spouse joins the therapy. It can also be problematic if a therapist takes sides on the basis of his or her personal bias about marriage, or to promote a political or social cause. If a therapist takes sides to promote feminism, for example, the husband may discredit the therapist by refusing to cooperate because the therapist is biased against him. Any intervention aimed at getting the husband to initiate a change will fail. The wife in this situation also may become annoyed with the therapist for alienating her husband. Perhaps she has just spent several months persuading him to attend marriage therapy with her, and then the therapist antagonizes her husband by espousing a social cause, a cause that the wife may view as unrelated to why she has come in.

One standard way of unbalancing couples within the approach offered here is to press the husband to go all out to demonstrate his love for his wife (Haley, 1996). The partners may come in upset with each other and neither wants to make the first move. If they are following the rule that the wife initiates and the husband responds, the husband never initiates affection. To break this pattern, and clarify how the husband feels, a therapist can intervene by insisting that the husband take the lead in demonstrating his love for his wife. The therapist pushes the husband to make the first move.

If the husband really does have doubts about the marriage, or is angry and resentful, these facts will come into focus as a consequence of the husband's being asked by a therapist to take the initiative. When he is put in this position, he has to play his hand. If he has doubts, he may or may not bring these up with the therapist, but what he must do is *decide* whether or not he really wants to warm up to his wife. If he does take the initiative, the wife's uncertainties about him are clarified and she will feel better. On the other hand, he may decide he is too angry with his wife to warm up to her and this issue then is brought out in the open. Sometimes, the partners separate. What is important is that by being asked by a therapist to take the initiative, the husband must clarify what he really wants and make his feelings explicit. An invisible man becomes visible.

The Rules

PRESENTING PROBLEM

Eric and Linda, a couple in their early 30s came to therapy requesting help with their marriage. Both had a college education and worked full time as professionals. They had been married for five years and had no children. The problem was that Eric had had an emotional affair. He had met a younger woman at his office who was single and distressed about personal issues, and he became her mentor. They met secretly for lunch, many times over several months. Eric counseled her and consoled her about her difficulties. They did not have a sexual relationship.

One day, Linda discovered a piece of paper with an unfamiliar phone number, and she dialed it. Eric's woman friend answered. Linda confronted Eric about the woman and Eric confessed he had been meeting with her in private. Linda's reaction was a deep feeling of insecurity. She wondered if Eric still loved her, if he wanted to be with her, and if he found her attractive. Linda constantly confronted Eric about the affair, thinking that it might still be active. Despite his repeated assurances that it was over, his lack of continued suspicious behavior, and his constant apologies, Linda's insecurities did not abate. Instead, she began to track Eric's whereabouts for every minute of the day, and called him constantly.

After several months of this, the couple started marital therapy with a female therapist. Her approach was to push Eric to express his sorrow for the affair and to take steps to make amends. She was very confrontational with him about the affair. This did not help Linda's insecurities, but instead exacerbated them. Although she herself was disturbed by Eric's actions, she did not want a therapist to alienate him. She was very protective of him. When the therapist did not back off, *Linda* fired her. Linda then sought a male therapist, on the assumption that Eric might relate better to a man, and they found their way to me.

When I saw them for the first time, it was apparent that Linda's insecurities were the main symptom. She had forgiven Eric, and trusted that he had stopped seeing his friend, a typical problem with affairs. Instead, what was remarkable was that although Eric reassured Linda daily that he found her attractive, that he loved her and he wanted to be with her, these reassurances had no effect on Linda's insecurities.

The general situation for this couple was that they had been married for several years but had no children and were reaching a stage of life at which there is pressure on couples to decide if and when they will have them. In our culture, we have few role models to help young couples know how to have a marriage without children. Obviously, they cannot look to their parents for this. As Haley describes it, this is a stage of life in which something is supposed to happen. If it does not, something else often happens instead. That something else can be the couple's establishing a business together or developing an intense interest that consumes some of the energy they would ordinarily put into being parents. Or one spouse might develop a problem such as depression, or one might have an affair. In this case, Eric had an emotional affair.

Three Problems

As I saw it, there were three problems. First, the partners' emotional closeness and distance were being regulated by Linda's insecurities. They were in a pattern in which Eric was attentive and affectionate when Linda was feeling insecure, and withdrew from her when she felt better. They were only close if Linda expressed her insecurities. Second, Eric's status was elevated when Linda needed reassurance. Linda became a needy female, and Eric had the status of being her helper. This was the same arrangement he was in with his needy woman friend. This made me wonder whether Eric might be one down in general in relation to Linda, and if Linda's insecurities were an attempt to correct this. This would explain why Linda became upset with the previous therapist. Finally, the third problem, related to the status issue, was that Eric was very contrite. He capitulated to Linda on anything she demanded. He was patronizing her. This made her too powerful, and him too mysterious.

Eric was not showing affection spontaneously. Linda had to become insecure to get it. And Eric capitulated on everything, making his true feelings a mystery. Because he always agreed with her, Linda assumed that Eric was withholding his real feelings and, therefore, was deceiving her. Eric's not showing affection spontaneously and his patronizing of Linda were the causes of her doubts about his feelings toward her. Eric was not showing his hand, and that made him invisible. The question was: Did this pattern of Eric's capitulating appear because he felt guilty about the affair, or was this pattern present before the affair?

I met with Eric privately and confronted him about his being so agreeable. He reacted to my confrontation by describing what he referred to as "*the Rules.*" He explained that approximately a year earlier, he had raised the question of having children with Linda. Having children was very important to Eric. He had discussed it with Linda before they were married, and she expressed a desire to have children as well. But when Eric raised the issue a second time, Linda said she was not ready. She did not want to give up her freedom. She wanted to travel and she wanted to save more money. Eric took these statements as demands with which he must comply. He felt as if Linda were laying down the law that he must take her on trips and save money before she would grant him a child. Instead of stating his position that he was ready for them to have children, and insisting that they try to achieve some sort of compromise, Eric gave in to Linda without further discussion. The couple disagreed on a very major issue, but instead of discussing and negotiating, Linda gave an intense response to Eric and Eric capitulated.

Eric's reaction to the idea of having to wait indefinitely before he and Linda would try to have children, and to what he considered her unreasonable demands to travel and save more money, was dejection. He felt he had no alternative but to carry out her orders, and this put him in a one-down position in the marriage. Fearing that Linda would respond with anger, Eric did not voice his feelings and so she was unaware of his resentment. Instead of discussing the issues with Linda, Eric withdrew. The problem was that Linda was too powerful. With this couple it was the husband, not the wife, who was one down, an arrangement that therapists miss if they have a bias that only women can be one down in a marriage.

Eric and Linda were following the pattern in which one spouse becomes intensely agitated about something. The other then capitulates without negotiating, and becomes resentful and withdraws. I have found that often the resentful spouse's withdrawal is sexual. In Eric's case, he withdrew emotionally. Typically, if it is the husband who is capitulating and resentful, when the wife confronts him about it, he denies he is upset. The capitulating spouse fears the intensity of the other spouse's reactions and so avoids discussions about potentially difficult issues. He is avoiding her intensity. Because no discussions take place, negotiating and compromising are not possible. The capitulating spouse, in this case, the husband, never gives his opinion on anything that might disturb his wife. He never states his position and so he becomes invisible. Linda was insecure because Eric indeed had withdrawn from her emotionally. But by patronizing her, he was denying that he was bothered about anything, and this intensified Linda's insecurities. From Eric's point of view, the quid pro quo became, "You can have your way on x, y, or z, but you are not going to have me emotionally."

It is important to understand that the spouse who capitulates ends up one down and the other spouse ends up as too powerful. One spouse capitulates to what he or she considers a unilateral decision by the other spouse. The capitulating spouse then loses power and becomes one down. One way he or she can then equalize the situation is by developing a symptom and, therefore, lowering his or her status. Equalizing power by lowering one's status is perhaps a common tactic when direct negotiations are not possible. When faced with a stubborn, intense spouse who is not open to discussing an issue, one can develop such symptoms as headaches, depression, or anxiety to do one's negotiating. Issues then are settled on the basis of one spouse's having a symptom. In the case of men who are one down, sexual or emotional withdrawal and/or finding another woman seem to be the symptoms of choice. But these choices result in a loss of status. The husband is either sexually dysfunctional, patronizing and spineless, or unfaithful. The capitulating spouse can be either the wife or the husband. Therapists who are on the warpath against "patriarchal" husbands are likely to miss an arrangement such as Eric and Linda's, in which the husband is the one who is one down. In fact, that is what had occurred with their previous therapist.

In Eric's case, his way of equalizing power by withdrawing and relating to another woman resulted in his losing status. His being exposed as unfaithful and having to give up the other woman, however, did not elevate his status, but lowered it further. The husband's status had to be elevated, not lowered, as it was in the previous therapy. Linda knew this. That is why *she* fired the previous therapist. Her insecurities could be thought of as her way of elevating Eric's status by putting him in the position of having to help her. She was sacrificing herself in the interest of helping him. This obviously was an unfortunate way for the couple to organize their relationship. It resulted in a paradox. By her providing him with a problem to solve, she was initiating the solution and this could not result in raising his status. The one-down spouse must raise his or her own status. To do this, the one-down spouse must take the initiative, not respond to the partner's initiative. To raise his or her own status, the one-down spouse must assert himself or herself.

When Eric explained "the Rules" to me, I chose to unbalance the couple by jumping on him for letting his wife get the better of him, not for his past misbehavior. I went after him for not being a man and stating his case, and for not insisting on some sort of compromise regarding children. I then went after him about his capitulating on everything. I asked him to name three things that Linda did with which he did not agree but gave in on. He easily came up with a list. I challenged his manhood and insisted that he discuss these concerns with Linda. The goal was not for him to force her to give in, but for him to name those issues with which he did not agree and insist that they reach some compromises.

I then had Linda join us. I took the position with the couple that the problem was not that Eric was an unfaithful husband, that problem was over. The problem was that Linda was getting her way on everything. Eric was not being open, but was just giving in without discussion. Far from being upset with the way I was defining the problem, Linda agreed with me and was relieved that I understood. She then explained that her father was that way with her mother and her mother was very unhappy. Linda did not want her marriage to be a repetition of her parents' marriage. She wanted to know how Eric really felt about various things and she could not tell because he always agreed with her.

I asked Eric to bring up the issue of children. Linda said that she was not ready for children. Eric stated that he wanted children soon. They discussed the subject at length, with both offering their ideas in detail. In my presence, after I had implied that Eric was a coward for not being more forthright, he was very open with Linda. The couple did not resolve the matter of children in this discussion, but I was not concerned about that. What was important was that they were discussing an important issue, one on which they disagreed, with no one getting killed. I encouraged the couple to have more discussions, and explained that they would have to reach some sort of compromise. I also explained to Linda that Eric had a list of several items on which he disagreed with her and that he would be bringing those items up for discussion and they would have to reach compromises on them as well.

The couple discussed the less important issues on Eric's list and began to reach some compromises. This provided them with practice at negotiating. As Eric asserted himself with his wife and insisted on compromises, his status in the marriage improved along with his self-esteem. By insisting on compromises, and not just capitulating, Eric was elevating his own status within the relationship. The couple did have some arguments about some of the issues, but unlike in the past, Eric did not just give in when Linda offered a different view. He did not want to have to face another male (myself) and admit that he was not man enough to state his case. By Eric's asserting his position on various problems, the couple was able to reach some compromises. Eric no longer was in a one-down position and he became less resentful. It was now possible to push him to be more affectionate.

Once the couple had reached a middle ground and Eric was feeling more positive about the situation, I raised the question of affection. I explained that Linda was having doubts about whether he truly loved her, and that he would have to find some way to help her resolve these doubts. To do this, he would have to initiate romantic gestures, not just respond when she was feeling insecure. Eric instantly came up with several ideas. It turned out that he had been very romantic in the past and knew exactly what Linda liked. He had stopped when he became upset with her, but now he realized he had to assert himself again. He began initiating little things that Linda liked, and this helped her immensely. As Eric began to initiate affection, Linda was reassured and her insecurities began to diminish.

Although Eric and Linda began to improve, they faced one last crisis when Eric had to take an extended business trip. This would be his first such trip since Linda had discovered his affair. She was very nervous; the trip would be a serious test of his trustworthiness. Eric and I discussed the problem and he decided that he needed to do something special to help her deal with his departure. Just before he left, he surprised her with a special night in a hotel. Linda was very touched and pleased. This gesture erased all her remaining doubts. The trip became their final turning point. He was faithful during his absence and Linda felt therapy was no longer needed. Therapy ended with the couple's deciding to have a baby. Linda came in to see me alone and explained that she had thought it over and felt the time was right. That was my last session with either of the couple. One year later, I received a card with a picture of a beautiful baby girl and two pleased parents.

Flushing Out the Truth

Gordon was in his late 40s when he sought therapy for the first time. He came alone for his initial visit. He had been married for 26 years, and he and his wife, Joan, had a 23-year-old son who lived on his own. Both Gordon and Joan were professionals, but Joan made more than Gordon and was considered by the couple to be the main breadwinner.

The problem was that Gordon had been having an affair for several months and was unsure whether or not he wanted to stay married to Joan. He said that he had strong feelings for his woman friend, and was not sure that he still loved his wife. He was reluctant to divorce her, however, citing the security his marriage provided. The more he saw his woman friend, the more tortured he became about what to do. He had become anxious and depressed and fearful that his wife would discover what he was doing.

He described his marriage as very unsatisfactory, his wife as emotionally and physically distant, and as having been so for years. He said Joan was not interested in affection and had refused any type of tender advances for so long that he had given up trying. The couple had had sex twice in the past two years. When he attempted to voice his dissatisfaction about the emotional distance, Joan would dismiss him by saying that he knew when he married her that she was not the affectionate type.

Gordon went on to explain that he could not assert himself with Joan about anything. If he did, she would become intensely angry and he would become tongue-tied and just drop whatever it was he was trying to bring up. Basically, Joan stifled Gordon, and he described himself as being in a one-down position. Because she stifled him, Gordon stated that pretty much everything went Joan's way. He survived the relationship by withdrawing from Joan.

The couple had lived separate lives for many years. Joan was active in the community, was on numerous boards, and was generally very busy outside the home. Gordon had a strong passion for playing the saxophone. He played in a small jazz group that performed in various pubs around town, and this kept him occupied in his free time. They had organized their marriage in such a way that they could live apart emotionally.

Gordon's current love interest was not his first. He had had affairs previously, and they had partly served to stabilize Gordon and Joan's distant arrangement. Their quid pro quo was that Joan could run the show at home, with Gordon defined as an underling, and then Gordon could withdraw and turn to other women and his music. In this arrangement, Gordon could give in to Joan on whatever she wanted, while he invested himself emotionally in doing other things. The truth was that Joan really did not want much emotionally from Gordon. She was just as invested elsewhere as he was.

The two were living parallel lives and although Gordon was dissatisfied with the arrangement, he rarely complained to Joan about it. He was certain that Joan was unaware of his unhappiness. At this point, he was also terrified to tell her that he was unhappy. Joan was not aware that Gordon had even come to therapy.

The problem now was that his current affair was different. This time, he had really become attached. Predictably, Gordon's woman friend was everything his wife was not. She listened to him, had similar interests, and was very affectionate.

I proposed to Gordon that he let me help him decide what to do. I postulated that his current anxiety and depression were attributable to his not knowing what decision to make and that the stakes seemed pretty high, no matter what he decided. I then explained how I might be most helpful to him. I took the position that after 26 years of marriage and a grown son, if he had doubts about what to do, my advice was to be conservative. That would mean not seeing his woman friend, and attempting to improve his marriage as a way to help himself figure out what to do. Put his best foot forward in his marriage and see if anything changed. If it did, he could stay in an improved marriage. If it did not, he could split, knowing that he had done all he could to improve things.

This is a standard approach in Strategic Therapy when a spouse is unsure about staying in a marriage. It is based on the belief that our field is not advanced enough for any of us to be able to predict whether or not a given couple can salvage a troubled marriage. Therefore, the best way to approach the problem is to attempt to commit the couple to improving things as a way to help them discover whether the relationship can be changed.

In this case, I knew in the initial session that I would want Joan to come in and that I needed a contract with Gordon that would satisfy both him and Joan. If Joan did come in, she could hardly be angry with Gordon for wanting to improve the marriage. The most she could do would be to say that she was satisfied with how things were already. The initial problem was that Gordon was terrified to even tell Joan that he was unhappy and wanted her to join him in marriage counseling.

I advised Gordon that, one way or another, eventually he would have to tell Joan something. He agreed. I proposed that he start by defying her on something small as a way of communicating to her that all was not well. He said he would try, but could not promise anything.

Gordon came in the next week with his chest puffing out and feeling very pleased with himself. He had managed to stand up to Joan on one small thing in the past week. On a Thursday evening, Joan paged him and instructed him to come home soon and to stop at the store on the way to pick up some items she needed. Gordon told her he was too busy to come home now, and that she would have to wait. Apparently this was a major breach of their quid pro quo. This refusal was not like Gordon at all. He said that he felt very empowered by this simple act. I asked about

Joan's reaction and what he reported was very interesting. He said Joan became very insecure. When she realized he had not fallen deathly ill, her only explanation for Gordon's behavior, she became very confused. She began to inquire whether Gordon was unhappy and if his feelings for her had changed. I took this reaction to indicate that Gordon had broken a long-standing, major implicit rule. It was also apparent that Joan's feelings for Gordon were deeper than he realized. This provided me with an opportunity to press Gordon to bring Joan into therapy. I told him to be honest with her about how unhappy he was, and to inform her that he had come to see me, and that I thought they should come in together the next time.

I also inquired about Gordon's woman friend. He had agreed in the last session that the best way for him to decide what he should do would be to focus on his marriage and to stop seeing her. He had not yet told this to her, however. I urged him to do so and played on his guilt to try to motivate him to cease seeing her. She had two small children and the children were becoming attached to Gordon. I reminded Gordon that it was not fair to these children to allow them to get attached to him in such an uncertain situation. The longer he continued to see their mother and them, the more attached they would become, and the more hurt they would be if he decided to reconcile with his wife. Gordon had not thought about this, and became upset with himself for letting it happen. He agreed for the sake of the children to talk to their mother before our next appointment and to call me and let me know how it went.

Gordon carried out the tasks of confronting both women. He told his woman friend that they would have to stop seeing each other until he could figure out what he wanted to do. She was upset, but Gordon stuck to his position. The more difficult talk was with Joan. He told her that he was very unhappy, felt totally neglected, had started therapy, and if nothing changed between them, he did not know whether he could stay married to her. Joan was devastated. She did not become angry; she became scared. She insisted on accompanying him to see me and wanted to know what she could do to change things.

The couple did come in together, and I began by seeing Joan alone. I asked her to describe their marriage, and she confirmed Gordon's account. She said they had been very distant for many years, that she was comfortable with the arrangement and assumed Gordon was also. When he confronted her earlier in the week, she realized how important he was to her and that she had indeed neglected him. She knew he wanted to be closer to her and admitted she had pushed him away. Her explanation was that she got tired of dealing with "a second child." She said that Gordon always deferred to her on everything. She had to make all of the decisions. If an important decision had to be made, when she asked for his opinion, he would say, "Whatever you think is best" or "I agree with what you are saying." Joan would then have to guess what Gordon really thought about the topic. She eventually lost both her respect for him and her romantic interest. I asked her how she typically responded if Gordon did assert himself, and she admitted that she had a temper, and that she probably did stifle him at times.

Gordon was avoiding what he anticipated would be an intense response from Joan if he offered his true views on anything, and this made him invisible. This resulted in Joan's having more power than she wanted. She did not want to make all of the decisions, with no input from Gordon. She had attempted in a number of ways over the years to get Gordon to assert himself. She tried to tone herself down, and to "allow" Gordon to have more say in things. This resulted in the paradox of Joan's attempting to equalize power by granting Gordon more power. Only someone in power can grant more power. This act cannot change the power imbalance. Only Gordon could do that by asserting himself and insisting that the situation change. I asked her permission to help Gordon to stand up to her more. She knew he would have to if the marriage were really going to be saved.

Joan was also very shaken by what Gordon had said to her. He had never threatened her with divorce. Gordon had equalized power by threatening to leave. This was only a temporary solution. She felt she had been distant from him for too long, and was very concerned that he had made up his mind to leave. She was very insecure about the situation and I was concerned that the threat of Gordon's leaving would intensify the situation in a way that would be counterproductive.

I brought the couple together and stated that I knew that Gordon was uncertain whether he wanted to stay in the marriage, and the problem at hand was for him to make a decision. I wanted this decision to be made based on the couple's putting their best foot forward to see if they could improve their marriage. To do this, Gordon would have to be willing to attempt to have positive times with Joan. The problem was that Gordon was reluctant to warm up to Joan, fearing that if he did, she would take it to mean that he had decided to stay. He did not want to do anything that would create false hopes for Joan. They were not in a context that was likely to lead to improvement, with Joan insecure about the situation and Gordon reluctant to initiate anything positive.

To change this, I proposed that the couple set a deadline for Gordon to make a decision. Between now and that date would be a trial period in which each would try to show affection to the other, with the understanding that no decision would be made either way until the arrival of the date they had set. Setting a date is a standard approach I learned from Haley for intervening in this type of situation. Along with setting a date, they would make an agreement that if they had a bad fight or underwent some difficult times during that period, they were still committed to staying together until that date. I hoped that setting a trial period would free Gordon to make positive moves toward Joan and would reassure Joan that Gordon was not just going to bolt at the first sign of trouble. They both liked this idea and agreed to a four-month trial period.

Over the next few sessions, the couple performed their pattern for me on countless occasions. An issue would be brought up, and Joan would get an intense look on her face and assert herself in a very determined way. Gordon would capitulate instantly, even though he did not agree. I would then have to press Gordon to give his true opinion on the topic. He was not asserting himself. Finally, I saw him alone and questioned him. He then described countless episodes over the years in which he had expressed his opinion and Joan had responded by becoming abusive.

"What do you do when she gets that way?" I asked.

"I just drop whatever the topic is, or agree with whatever she is saying," he responded.

"Have you ever told her just to knock it off, not to treat you that way?" I inquired.

He looked dumbfounded, as if this were not possible. He obviously had never done so. I told him that I thought the appropriate thing for him to do if Joan were to become abusive would be to stand up for himself and to tell her he was not going to put up with that kind of treatment. I said, "The next time she does that, tell her to cut it out!"

Two weeks later, a major breakthrough occurred. Gordon described a discussion he and Joan were having in which Joan got the intense look in her eyes and started to become abusive. Gordon responded by calmly telling her in a nonhostile manner to back off and settle down. If she could not discuss the matter calmly, the discussion was over. I asked how Joan reacted to this. Gordon said she respected his request, and the two went on to have a reasonable discussion. Gordon said after he had done this he had felt like a new man. It was as if he had slain a dragon. In their 26 years of marriage, Gordon had never done anything like this. He said for the first time in their relationship, he felt like her equal. I was impressed not only with how Gordon had asserted himself in a nonhostile way, but also with how Joan had reacted by respecting his request.

After this episode, Gordon said he felt better about the prospects of improving the marriage, and over the next two months, they focused on spending more time with each other, going on dates, and even taking a short trip together. During this period, Joan had some relapses in which she was abusive. But each time she relapsed, Gordon brought it to her attention and she checked herself. Gordon told me that he never thought his relationship with Joan could go as well as it had during the past two months. Even with these positive times, however, he was still unsure what his decision would be.

As their decision date approached, Gordon asked to see me privately. He told me that Joan had been behaving irrationally, and her actions were beginning to upset him. I asked him what he meant by irrational behavior. He said that she would become very upset by nonsensical things. When he gave the following example, it became clear to me what was going on. Several nights earlier, Joan had been perturbed because Gordon did not "read her mind." For years, the couple's bedtime ritual had been for Joan to go to bed by herself and read for a half an hour, while Gordon remained downstairs and flipped through all the cable channels. After checking out all 70 channels, Gordon would go to bed and the couple would go to sleep.

On this particular night, Joan announced the fact that she was going upstairs, something she did not normally do. Gordon did not think anything of it and followed his usual routine. About 10 minutes later, Joan bellowed down, "Aren't you going to come up?" Gordon instantly turned off the TV and rushed upstairs. Joan was agitated because Gordon did not come to bed with her when she told him that she was going upstairs. She wanted them to spend some time together. When Gordon realized this, he said, "OK, that's a good idea." Joan then said, "It's too late now!" Gordon was very annoyed with her and mystified by the whole scenario.

It was clear to me, however, that what Joan wanted was for Gordon to join her upstairs because he wanted to spend time with her, not because she had to insist that he come up. This made me think that Gordon was not initiating affection with Joan. I asked him about it and he admitted that if they became affectionate, even in the slightest way, it was not he who made the first move. I explained to him that in a context in which Joan was unsure as to whether or not Gordon was going to stay in the marriage, and with the decision date looming, his lack of initiative could be very worrisome to her. I explained that Joan was probably feeling very insecure at this point and that the best way to calm her down and reassure her would be for him to initiate affectionate gestures.

Gordon then admitted that he did not know whether he could do so. He said that after 26 years of emotional abuse, he was not sure that he still loved Joan. He had been willing to stop seeing his woman friend, and to set up a trial period during which he would not leave no matter what happened, but that was all he could give. He could respond if she initiated affection, but inside he was not enthusiastic about warming up to Joan again. On the other hand, he also admitted that he was still unsure what his decision would be at the end of the trial period.

It is typical that when a date is set, as in this case, as the date approaches, the crucial issues will be flushed out. Gordon was willing to play along, but he was not willing to show his hand. He could respond with affection if Joan initiated it. But apparently he was just pretending. The question was whether too much water had gone under the bridge for Gordon to forgive Joan and start over. Although he agreed to attempt to improve the marriage, his heart was not in it, and he was revealing himself by only responding to Joan's initiating affection, and not initiating it himself. Because he continued to be unsure about his decision, I urged him to be more demonstrative with Joan and to note how he reacted. Pushing himself to be more affectionate would help him to know what he should do about the marriage.

At the next session, I started with Gordon alone and asked him what he had tried. He said he had really made an effort to initiate affection with Joan, but he just could not bring himself to do it. By trying very hard to do this, and not being able to, he had realized that he wanted out of the marriage. After all the years of what he considered emotional neglect and abuse, he could not forgive her. He had made his decision. My giving Gordon the directive to be affectionate helped him to clarify his position. By being put in the position of having to woo Joan, he was forced to decide. The truth had been flushed out. I asked him if he had told Joan, and he said that he had told her he was leaning toward leaving. I brought Joan in and she was very upset. She said that she had suspected that Gordon wanted out of the marriage because during the trial period, she always had to be the one to cuddle up to Gordon, or to take his hand, or to put her arm around him. He never initiated any of these things. Joan had realized exactly what was going on.

With Joan in the room, Gordon was very sheepish, but he

held to his position that he thought the marriage was over. In one last attempt to salvage the situation, I suggested that they spend the weekend together. After 26 years together, if they did split up, they deserved one last fling. The weekend would be followed by their separating for one week with no contact, not even telephone calls. During their week apart, Gordon would think seriously about the situation to make sure about what he wanted. I was not convinced that his decision was final. I wanted to put him through an ordeal to help him make sure, and to convince Joan that this was really what he wanted. The couple agreed to both the weekend together and the week apart.

After they did both, Gordon held to his position that he wanted out. Two weeks later, he moved in with his brother. The couple initiated divorce proceedings and began the process of splitting up. As time went on, Gordon reported that he was feeling better about himself than he had in years. He had no regrets about leaving and was certain that divorce was the right solution. Joan was unhappy about it, and was not ready to give up on attempting to salvage the marriage, but accepted that Gordon was determined to go through with divorce.

In both of the examples offered here, the husbands were in a one-down relationship with their wives. They were unable to assert themselves and to insist on negotiating on important issues. They were afraid to do so, fearing intense reactions from their wives. Instead of asserting themselves, they capitulated on whatever their wives demanded. They then became resentful and withdrew sexually, or emotionally, or both. They just disappeared. The problem was getting the husbands to assert themselves and to insist on negotiating. In one case, this led to the husband's reconnecting with his wife and the couple stayed together. In the other example, this led to the husband's admitting that he wanted out of the marriage. In both cases, unbalancing was used to get the husband to assert himself. I joined with the husband and challenged him.

4

Pregnant Fathers

After giving birth to her first child, a young woman fell into a deep depression. She and her husband had been married for six years. They both had careers and had planned to have the child. The woman's plan had been to take time off from her job at first, and then to work part-time while the child was an infant. She was diagnosed with postpartum depression and put on Prozac. She did not respond well to the medication and so was referred to a therapist, who worked with her individually. This did not seem to help. When it was time for her to return to work, the woman's mother moved in temporarily to help with the baby and with the young woman's depression. After a few months, the depression still did not lift. The professionals changed their diagnosis to major depression and explained that the woman would have to stay on her medication indefinitely. She became suicidal and was hospitalized. Her baby was then taken in by her sister. While she was in the hospital, it was decided to apply electroshock therapy.

The woman was the focus of all of the interventions by both professionals and her family. What was missed was the husband. The wife was the one who was diagnosed and put on medication. The wife was the one hospitalized and the one who received the shock treatments.

Years later, the couple divorced. At that time, the woman confessed to her family that her husband had not wanted the baby, and had had an affair just before the child's birth. The affair remained ongoing throughout the woman's hospitalization. While depressed, however, despite her anguish over her husband's behavior, the woman was protective of him and did not want to disclose the affair. Finally, the husband gave up his woman friend and his wife recovered. The woman had the diagnosis. The husband had the problem. The professionals had missed the whole thing.

THE COUVADE

Failure to adjust to life-cycle changes has long been viewed as a strong influence on the etiology of symptoms (Haley, 1973). A life-cycle stage of particular interest regarding the topic of invisible men is that of pregnancy and the birth of a couple's first child. This is a time when the pregnant mother can develop symptoms and become the focus of interventions. Fathers are overlooked. This is not so in many tribal cultures, however. Often, a tribal tradition will supply a family with a ritual designed to help it to adjust to life-cycle changes. With regard to childbirth, anthropologists, such as Margaret Mead and Gregory Bateson in the South Seas and George Gorer in the Himalayas, began observing birth rituals involving the fathers that were remarkable in their complexity and were widespread among tribal cultures. E. B. Tylor (1865) named the rituals "couvade," a French word meaning to brood over. Once these rituals attracted the attention of other anthropologists, they were observed in tribal cultures on every continent of the globe (Hall, 1989).

To appreciate the couvade ritual's complexity, and more important, its possible social function, it is worth examining a specific example. When his wife had not menstruated after three successive moon cycles, the New Guinea hunter withdrew from the males of his tribe, ceasing all hunting, fishing, and other male activities. He began to make his own clothing that he wore specifically for the period of his wife's pregnancy. He wore earrings identical to those of his wife and a special headdress made of feathers from birds associated with nesting. He visited his wife's family and avoided his own.

Through the fifth month of the pregnancy, he gathered food and hunted specifically to stockpile provisions for the baby. Then he ceased going out, relying on gifts of food from his wife's family. He devoted his time to building a hut for himself, close to that of his wife. In the final weeks, he and his wife slept apart, with the husband praying and chanting. In some rituals, during the final weeks of the mother's pregnancy, the father must mimic the pregnant mother's dress, and even go through symbolic labor.

This extensive ritual, which focuses on the father and encompasses his wife's entire pregnancy, can be considered to have many social functions. Typically, it is enacted during the birth of a man's first child. The obvious aim is to prepare the man for becoming a father. Throughout the ritual, he is demonstrating his commitment to the mother and the coming child. By mimicking her, he is put in sympathetic and compassionate contact with her. During the course of the pregnancy, the father is very active and focused on the pregnancy. By focusing on his rituals, the father is distracted from any doubts he may have about becoming a father and from any temptations to do something inappropriate.

What is also impressive is that the ritual prescribes the role of every tribal individual in relation to the expectant father. His relationships with his own family, his wife's family, and his fellow tribesmen are all governed by the couvade. He withdraws from his own family, but this is expected, and so his family will not be disturbed by his behavior. He also withdraws from his male friends, but again, they will be supportive of his withdrawal. The ritual ensures that the expectant father will not be placed in any conflicting triangles regarding the pregnancy among any of his intimate relationships.

Contrast this ritual with the stereotypical way in which our culture handles this life transition. It appears that an expectant father can react to a pregnancy in any of three ways (Richman, 1978). He can deny the pregnancy, possibly even abandoning the mother and/or connecting with another woman. Or he can regard the pregnancy as the mother's responsibility, and place himself as a peripheral participant. He may help if asked. Or he can establish a special bond with the fetus and share the pregnancy experience. In our culture, it appears that the first two choices predominate. When a woman becomes pregnant, it is most likely she who consults with outside experts, conducts research, charts progress, plans projects, attends baby showers, and takes classes. Throughout the pregnancy, the mother is totally involved with the pregnancy. The father may be involved to a great degree, or not at all. We have no specific ritual or custom that focuses the expectant father so intensively on the mother's pregnancy. In our culture, when a woman becomes pregnant, what is the father supposed to do? His level of participation is essentially left up to each individual set of parents to work out, with no clear cultural guidelines.

Lacking a clear tradition, this can be a time when either parent can feel tremendous pressure. Pregnancy forces both mother and father to face issues concerning their relationship that can result in one or both acting strange. If they are married, either one may fear the increased commitment to the marriage, especially if he or she already has doubts. The father may fear new responsibilities, and feel left out and ignorant of the process and lost regarding his role. In light of this, it is not surprising that men can behave erratically during this time, and exhibit a multitude of symptoms, such as having an affair, abusing alcohol, or distancing themselves from the prospective mother at a crucial juncture in their relationship. Without a powerful ritual such as the couvade to focus the father on the pregnancy, define his role, and govern his behavior, he is free to struggle with this difficult period in any number of problematic ways. If the expectant mother is counting on his participation, erratic behavior by him can contribute to the symptoms experienced by her.

Another consequence of having no customary ritual is that professionals become overly focused on the mother during this period. The father becomes invisible. If the mother develops problems during or just after pregnancy, such as postpartum depression, she is the subject of the diagnosis and the treatment. The father's possible complicity is missed.

In extreme cases, this response to postpartum symptoms, by family and professionals, of overly focusing on the mother can exacerbate the problem. If the mother is hospitalized, or prevented from caring for her baby herself, at a time when bonding with the child is crucial, her symptoms can worsen and create a spiraling deterioration. The issue that is often missed is that the wife will protect the husband by becoming symptomatic herself. The professionals then focus on the wife as having postpartum symptoms, and miss the fact that the problem is really related to a father who is having difficulties.

Rhonda Burnaugh learned this lesson early in her nursing career when a pregnant woman was admitted to the hospital ward because of excessive vomiting. She could not keep any food down, was dehydrated, and had to be fed intravenously. At one point during the woman's hospitalization, her husband flirted with Rhonda, which aroused her suspicions. She took the husband aside and began asking him about his marriage. He explained that he did not want the baby, and that he had agreed that they have a child because his wife was adamant about it. Since his wife became pregnant, he had been distancing himself from her emotionally, and even began to have an affair. The wife was admitted to the hospital with the symptoms, but the husband was the one who was struggling with the pregnancy.

After learning about this couple and their problems, Rhonda began to look out for other pregnant women who came to the hospital with similar symptoms. Over the next few months, two more women were admitted for the same type of problems, and Rhonda interviewed their husbands. In both cases, the husbands were ambivalent about the pregnancy and were having affairs. In all three cases in which pregnant wives were admitted to the hospital with vomiting as a symptom, their husbands were having affairs. The husbands were having problems, and they were making their wives sick to their stomachs.

The fact that so many diverse tribes have developed an elaborate ritual for *fathers* at this life-cycle juncture should alert us to the father's crucial role during this period, and his complicity if the mother develops symptoms. Like the couvade, if a mother has symptoms during or just after pregnancy, the approach offered here focuses on the father. We assume that if the wife is having symptoms, it is often in response to the father's struggling with the pregnancy, or behaving erratically or dispassionately. Also like the couvade, if the wife is having difficulty, the father is given a dramatic ritual as one remedy to help correct the problem. These therapeutic rituals not only give the father some task to do in relation to his pregnant wife, but they also indirectly prescribe the roles of the extended family and the father's peers with regard to the pregnancy and new birth.

THE COACH

A couple in their mid-20s came in to therapy. They had been married for four years and had no children. Both were college graduates and had full-time jobs. In addition to his work, the husband, John, coached Little League soccer and hockey, a sport for almost every season of the year. When he was not out coaching, he was at home watching soccer or hockey on TV so he could pick up coaching tips. He had three television sets so he could watch three games simultaneously.

Presenting Problem

Amazingly, John's wife, Julie, had adjusted to his obsession with sports. The problem that brought them into therapy was that Julie had just found out that she was pregnant and John was not enthusiastic about their having a child. He wanted to have children eventually, but not now. He was very concerned that they could not afford it at this time. Julie would have to leave her full-time job and he did not see how they could do without her salary. Also, having a child now would compromise his career goal of obtaining a college coaching position, a goal that, as he adamantly pointed out, his wife knew was important to him when they first got married. He was also afraid that he was not ready to be a father. And worst of all, the child was not due until October, and that would be the middle of the soccer season. The child's birth would disrupt the whole season.

Julie was very upset by John's wavering about having the baby. She wanted a child and thought all of his concerns were unimportant. She felt they would work out the finances somehow. Not surprisingly, she was rather disgusted with John's concern that the birth of the child would interfere with the soccer season. She was determined to have this child, and was dragging him in to see me so that I could correct his mistaken attitude.

Wanting to understand whether the problem involved the extended family, I asked if they had discussed the situation with their respective parents. They had not. They wanted to wait until they had decided how they were going to handle it. This seemed wise on their part, keeping a boundary around themselves and not including the relatives in a way that could put the entire extended family in an uproar.

My problem was with whom I should be in a coalition. If I sided with the husband, the wife would instantly fire me. If I sided with the wife regarding having the child, I could cause even greater problems. If I did side with the wife and the husband went along with having the child, it would be because he was pressured by his wife and a professional, not because he actually wanted the child. The wife did not understand how her pressuring him would intensify her own problem. She was creating a situation with which she herself ultimately would be unsatisfied. She wanted her husband to *want* to have the child. For this to happen, the husband would have to reach that decision on his own, without being pressured by anyone.

I asked John if he had any coaching colleagues who were married and had children. He said that he did have two coaching mentors who were in their 40s and had children. I ended the first session suggesting to John that he discuss the situation with his mentors and get their advice. This seemed safe as it would not result in problems with the larger families and might result in John's changing his position on his own.

John did seek the advice of the other coaches and the couple returned for the next interview transformed. Both of them had given him the same advice. They both told him that he would never be ready to have his first child, and that he would always worry that he and his wife could not afford one. But they reassured him that when his wife had the baby, he would fall in love with his child and wonder how he could ever have doubted that they should have it. They also told him that it was normal for him to wonder if he would be a good father. To Julie's delight, John took their advice to heart and changed his mind about having the child.

Both John and Julie were pleased with the situation and did not think they needed to return to see me. I was pleased that they were satisfied and that after only two sessions, I could keep my reputation with the HMO as a miracle worker.

Relapse

Four months later, Julie called me and told me that she wanted to come in alone. She was very depressed. I agreed to see her, and when she came in, she looked terrible. She said, "I am having a baby, both my husband and I want the child, and I should be excited, but instead I am very depressed." She had not worked in over a week, but stayed in bed all day and could barely function. If she did get out of bed, she would not shower or put on make-up, but would remain all day in her grungiest robe. She had already been to a physician, who had put her on antidepressant medication.

I knew the couple's situation and was not buying that she did not know why she was upset. I was assuming that she was protecting John by saying she did not know the reason for her depression. She was distracting the professionals' attention from John's complicity in the problem. The doctor who had medicated her had already fallen for this. It was easy to see why, however. If one focused solely on her symptoms, and not on her situation, she would easily have met the criteria for a major depressive episode.

I asked Julie about her and John's daily routine prior to her becoming depressed. She said that they both would get up early and go to work. She would get home around 6:00 P.M. and would then have to do housework. John did not get home until 9:00 or 10:00 P.M., or, if he did get home early, he would have to watch sports to get his coaching ideas. With this schedule, he, of course, could not be expected to help around the house. On weekends

John was just as unavailable. He was gone most of the time, coaching or watching films of the games he had just coached.

After listening to all of this, I asked Julie one question. "Where in that routine is there room for anyone to take care of an infant?"

Julie responded by breaking down and crying. She admitted she was very worried about that. In fact, that was why she was depressed. She was afraid to suggest to John that she cut back to part-time work because John was so concerned about finances. She could not ask him to cut back on coaching, his life's passion. She also explained that his father was a coach and his mother was "superwife." Somehow, in spite of John's father being away all of the time, his mother managed to take charge of the house and to raise three children with no help from her husband. Julie feared that John had the same expectations of her and she did not see how she could meet them.

The problem, as I saw it, was that John was saying that he wanted a child, but he was not acting like it. He was not making any preparations for a child, and this was behaviorally communicating ambivalence about having a baby. He had not changed his routine in the slightest way that would communicate to Julie that he was preparing for the arrival of a new baby. I assumed that this was the cause of her depression. Because John was acting as if there were no baby on the way, Julie was not sure that he really wanted the child.

Adding to all of this was the problem that Julie believed John was not open to verbal negotiations with her regarding the changes required to accommodate a child. Her depression could be thought of in part as having a function in the couple's relationship. When faced with a husband who is not open to negotiating, one can become depressed and force the issue. Julie's depression was resulting in her not working. If John would not negotiate for changes in the couple's routine that would accommodate a child, Julie's depression would negotiate for them. Her depression would force her to stay home and create a routine whereby she could be home with a baby. Unfortunately, this way of dealing with the issues could be fraught with a multitude of obvious problems.

After listening to Julie's story, and privately developing the above hypothesis, I ended the session by asking Julie to return in two days with John.

A Therapeutic Couvade

Two days later, John and Julie came in together. I asked John to describe his wife's condition. He said that she was very depressed and was barely functioning. Every morning, he would get up, take a shower, and get ready for work. Julie would stay in bed. Before he left for work, he would attempt to get her off to her job. He tried to be encouraging, but that did not help. Lately, he was feeling frustrated and was becoming angry with her. That did not help either. The more he attempted to motivate her to get up and get going, the worse she got. To make matters worse, despite Julie's deteriorating condition, after struggling with her in the morning, John would go about his daily routine as if nothing were wrong.

After listening to this, I got John alone and asked him to tell me honestly whether or not he really did want this child. He said emphatically that he did. "You are not acting like it," I responded. He became confused. I explained that having a child would be a life-altering event, requiring major changes in his and Julie's daily routines and requiring many preparations by both of them. One or both of them might have to change their work schedules. Julie might have to work part-time, or not at all for a while. He might have to cut back on his coaching. He said he knew something would have to change, but that was months away, and he was not thinking about it now. It had not occurred to him to discuss any of those things with his wife, or how he might be involved with her regarding her pregnancy. With no clear cultural tradition governing his conduct during the period of Julie's pregnancy, John was free to act as if she were not pregnant. I explained to him that he was conducting his life as if his wife were not pregnant and that might be very confusing to her.

Privately, I was thinking that Julie, because of John's initial reluctance, was still uncertain about John's true feelings regarding having the child. She might be waiting for him to initiate discussions about how he might be involved with the pregnancy now, or about changes that would be required related to having the child. For example, if he really wanted the child, he might spontaneously bring up getting a nursery prepared, or do something else that would show that he was preparing for a child. He was not initiating such discussions, and this was exacerbating Julie's doubts. Julie already knew that if she brought up the topic, John would say that he wanted the child. The problem was that he was not backing up his words with any kind of behavior. If Julie had to initiate a talk about it, she would then interpret his responses to her inquiries as patronizing her. John needed to take some action that would communicate his sincerity about wanting the child, not just respond if Julie brought up the topic.

The first order of business, however, was to focus directly on Julie's depression. I told John that I had something for him to do, and if he were willing to do it, it would get Julie activated again very quickly. He was interested. I told him it would require a sacrifice by him. He said OK. I explained that he would have to stay home from work. He agreed. I wanted him to do something dramatic, which would demonstrate his concern about how she was feeling. I thought it needed to be dramatic because Julie's problem was very dramatic. I wanted it to be something that would change their current pattern of John's trying to get Julie up and out of bed, and her resisting him and getting worse. This is typical of a couple where one spouse is depressed. The nondepressed spouse attempts to motivate the depressed spouse and the depressed spouse reacts by feeling that the depression is not being taken seriously. The depressed spouse then becomes more depressed to prove that he or she is really depressed.

Most important, as with the couvade, I wanted this to be a ritual that would demonstrate John's commitment to Julie and to them as a couple. I wanted John to do something that would put him into sympathetic and intimate contact with Julie's dilemma.

"Today is Wednesday," I said to John. "Tomorrow morning, when you awaken, if Julie is still depressed, you are *not* to take a shower and get ready for work. Nor are you to attempt to motivate her to get out of bed and go to work. Instead, when you wake up, you are to put on your rattiest sweat clothes and get into bed with her. Tell her that if she is so unhappy, you cannot possibly function and go to work. If she is this upset, you are upset also, and will have to stay in bed with her all day."

I instructed him to stay in bed with her for as long as she stayed in bed depressed. If that took one day, OK; if it took nine months, then that is how long it would take. He would have to take time off from work and suspend his coaching until she improved. I told him it was possible that this could take a long time, but I really doubted that she would stay in bed very long if he did this. He agreed to do it.

This ritual would be the opposite of what John was currently doing. Instead of his nagging her to get out of bed and then just going about his day as if nothing were wrong, he would cancel everything. As with the couvade, he would withdraw from his male world to be with his wife. I assumed that giving him a ritual that would allow him to demonstrate his willingness to sacrifice work and coaching in order to help her would erase any doubts she might have of his sincerity about changing their lives to accommodate a new child. Also, I thought that the last thing Julie would want would be for John to sacrifice his whole day to be stuck in bed with her. Finally, I thought that if John really did have doubts about having the child, the prospect of having to give up everything to deal with a depressed wife would be far worse than any changes he might have to make to accommodate a new baby.

I also gave John one last directive. I suggested that it might be a good idea, while he and Julie were in bed together, for him to bring up the subject of what changes they were going to have to make to prepare for having their child. I emphasized that I wanted *him* to bring this up, and not to wait for her to do so. John was asked to negotiate directly with Julie about this issue and to be prepared to sacrifice something to fit having a baby into his life.

Follow-up

The couple went home, and the next morning, John carried out the plan. Julie was shocked. They did discuss the changes they would need to make to have the baby. John agreed that it would be wise for Julie to cut back to part-time work, and for him to eliminate coaching soccer. He would continue to coach hockey, since coaching college hockey was his main goal. John and Julie stayed in bed together on Thursday and Friday and all weekend. On Monday, Julie got up and went to work. John became more involved with Julie during the pregnancy, going with her to the doctor, and taking classes with her. Julie recovered. That fall I received a card with a picture of a baby boy.

Haley's Case

The above case demonstrates difficulties that can occur if the father is reluctant about the couple's having a child, or if the mother is concerned that the father is reluctant. Both John and Julie wanted to be married, but John was unsure that he was ready for them to have a child. Another possible problem is that one of the partners is ambivalent about the marriage itself. In this situation, the wife's becoming pregnant forces the issue. Having doubts about wanting to be with your spouse is a difficult problem that becomes more intense when the wife gets pregnant. A child cements the marriage. That is real trouble if you are not sure you want to be married in the first place. The following case is an example of this dilemma. In the 1950s, Jay Haley had a small private practice, and a psychiatrist friend referred a woman to him who was constantly crying (Haley, 1973, 1994). The psychiatrist had been seeing the client for about three months. She had started to cry when she gave birth to her first child. Initially, Haley assumed the husband was struggling with the couple's having their first child. As the case unfolded, however, he began to suspect that the wife was having doubts about the marriage.

The young mother had begun to cry so uncontrollably after the baby was born that her husband took her into his mother's home so that his mother could help her take care of the baby. While living with her mother-in-law, the mother just sat and cried. She could not do anything. She said, "I can't take care of the baby. I can't do it." The husband would ask her to feed the baby. She would respond, "I can't feed the baby."

She came to Haley and cried. She could cry 10 to 12 hours a day. At the second interview, Haley had the father in and asked him about the problem. During the interview, the woman stopped crying to correct her husband's account of the problem, which was one way to get her to stop crying.

Haley learned from the man that the two were married, owned a home, and that this was their first child. When the wife began to be depressed and to cry, they closed up the house and moved in with his family. His mother then took over caring for the baby. The wife said that when her husband came home from work, he did not ask her about the baby:

"He goes to his mother, because his mother knows about the baby. I can't take care of the baby."

The husband told Haley that he only spent 15 or 20 minutes a day with his wife, because she cried all the time.

Haley asked them, "Do you plan ultimately to go back to your own house?"

They both said, "Certainly, we're going to go back."

Then Haley said, "Well, it's just a matter of when."

This was on a Monday. Haley asked, "Could you move back into your house by Thursday?"

"I guess we could," said the husband.

"We couldn't possibly move back into that house by Thursday!" shouted the wife.

"It hasn't been painted, it's been closed up. We've got to arrange everything for the baby. We didn't fix up a room for the baby."

As with the previous couple, this couple had made no preparations for the arrival of the baby, a signal that one or both might have been ambivalent about having the child, or about the marriage itself.

Haley said he thought the couple could move in by Thursday, and possibly even by Wednesday.

The wife told Haley, "We couldn't possibly go in there before Friday."

They got busy putting the house in order, and they moved in. Haley quickly got them back to a more normal routine in which the wife, not the husband's mother, was taking care of the baby. They moved back into their home, but the wife continued to cry.

Haley decided to make a home visit. The wife was still crying, but she was doing what she had to do. Haley then gave the husband a ritual. He was to stay home for two weeks, to take care of his wife and the new baby and make sure that things were OK. He was asked to make a sacrifice that would demonstrate his sincerity and commitment to their having a child. The husband agreed and took the time off.

A few days after the husband went back to work, Haley got a call from the wife. She said she was unhappy, crying, depressed, and wanted to talk. Haley said, "I only have time to come for lunch, and I am accustomed to very good lunches. I expect you to provide me with a good one." Haley got her busy making a good lunch. To do that would take some time. She would have to be active. She would have to worry what she should serve him, and so on. She would have to pull herself together. Activity often helps a depressed client pull out of a depression.

Haley arrived, and the woman was crying as she held the baby. It was a happy, cheerful baby, smiling while the mother sat there with tears running down her cheeks. Haley chatted with her for an hour. Then they had lunch and Haley departed. That was it. The next day, the wife stopped crying. She called a friend. She began to go to the grocery store. Haley treated her as though she did not need a therapist, she just needed to get organized. He came over for lunch, and she got organized being a proper hostess.

Haley never did find out why she was crying. He assumed that the husband was shaken by the pregnancy. Perhaps he suspected that his wife was unsure whether she wanted to stay with him and this upset him. By putting him in charge and having him take time off to be able to help his wife, Haley helped the husband pull himself together. Like the couvade, he was given a ritual that focused him on his wife and new baby.

But Haley also suspected that the wife questioned the marriage to the point that she was crying. She might have felt trapped. However, she apparently made a decision to stay in the marriage and got herself back to normal. But she kept her feelings about the marriage private, and Haley did not press her.

Haley assumed that the husband was shaken, and that the wife could have a baby and take care of it on her own, and would if her husband was handled well and involved properly in the intervention. Haley first had to get the couple back to what in their culture would be a normal arrangement: the child's mother staying home and caring for the baby and the husband supporting them. To do this, the mother-in-law had to be taken out of the child-care role and the mother helped to behave more competently with the baby. As with the couvade, an intervention had to be offered that prescribed everyone's role in relation to the new baby. Underscoring the importance of this, at one point, the mother-in-law said, "I'm not sure my grandchild should be raised by a woman in this condition."

Most important, the husband was given a task as part of the remedy to help the wife recover. The task focused him intensively on his wife and child, requiring him to pull himself together, and perhaps convincing his wife that she should stay with him. For inspiration regarding what interventions to offer a husband whose wife is symptomatic during this stage of life, a therapist need only look to the couvade.

5

Symptomatic Wives and Their Lost Husbands

The following three sections offer detailed accounts of therapies with very dysfunctional and/or disturbed clients. The clients are married women and their symptoms range from chronic and severe psychosis, to totally debilitating psychosomatic symptoms, to chronic and serious eating disorders. All three cases were approached with the assumption that the client's symptoms were partly the result of a quid pro quo between the couple. We assumed that the marital situation required the clients to be severely symptomatic. The couples were following the rule that the wife must have the symptoms and pretend that the husband is competent and healthy.

Regarding symptomatic wives, it appears as if the husbands of phobic wives have received the most attention in the literature. The main issue for our purposes is: If husbands are complicit in their wives' symptoms, what should be done about it? The problem has been presented as the husband having problems of his own that are masked by his wife's agoraphobia. Mittelmann (1958) apparently was the first to speculate about this. Mittelmann pointed out complementary patterns between the spouses in which the husband's confidence was bolstered by the sick wife's dependence. The classic example is shown by work done by William Fry (1962) at the Mental Research Institute. Fry reported that the husbands of agoraphobic wives, upon close inspection, had a history of symptoms almost identical to those of their spouses, but the husband's symptoms abated after the wife's problems developed. Fry also reported that, in some cases, the onset of the wife's symptoms correlated with a negative change in the life of the husband. He found that the wife's symptoms seemed to be serving the function of helping the husband, and of keeping the couple united. He described the situation as one of dual control, in which both husband and wife restricted each other's freedoms. He described a quid pro quo for agoraphobia.

The wife becomes panic stricken when she leaves the house. She may only be able to go to certain locations without suffering severe anxiety. In the quid pro quo way of thinking, it would be assumed that the marriage contract between the couple requires the wife to have agoraphobia. One question with a couple like this might be: What is the trade-off? Why is this symptom required? Such a symptom might develop if the husband were jealous and insecure if his wife went out in public. If this issue were too hot to discuss aloud, or if the husband was too uncomfortable to talk openly about it, the wife could develop agoraphobia as a way of silently accommodating the husband's insecurity. Explicitly, she would not be going out because of her agoraphobia, not because her husband was insecure. She would be protecting him by calling attention to herself. Professionals might then become concerned about her, not her husband. He would be invisible.

In exchange for her staying home, the husband might have to call his wife constantly to make sure she was OK. He might also have to come straight home after work every day to check on her. The contract would be: The wife would allow the husband to restrict her because of his jealousy, and not to speak aloud of the jealousy, in exchange for the husband's restricting his activities as well. Like the wife, the husband would have to restrict his activities on the basis of the wife's agoraphobia. She could become panic stricken at any time. He might be needed by her. This contract defines the wife as having a problem and the husband as the wife's helper (Grove & Haley, 1992).

Several researchers have documented the pathology of husbands of agoraphobic wives and the impediment this poses to the treatment of the wife's agoraphobia. Agulink (1970) studied 50 married phobic patients and suggested that the spouse of the patient was "fortified" by the dependence of the phobic spouse. Goodstein came to similar conclusions in the treatment of four phobic wives, one with a "contamination" phobia, one with a specific phobia, and two with generalized agoraphobia. In all four cases, the husband was found to be seriously symptomatic, and in three of the cases, it was concluded that the husband's participation in the treatment was necessary (Goodstein & Swift, 1977). Hafner treated 36 married female agoraphobic patients over a three-year period. He applied a standard four-day intensive outpatient behavioral treatment program. He reported that 20% were married to what he described as abnormally jealous men. In all of these cases, the husband's jealousy adversely influenced his wife's response to treatment, and most interesting, all of these husbands became symptomatic in response to improvement by their wives (Hafner, 1977). Hafner also found that in 50% of 33 agoraphobic wives, the husbands reacted negatively to their wives' improvement (Hafner, 1983). Hafner concluded that the husband's reaction to improvement was the main predictor of the success of treatment (Hafner, 1977, 1983). It appears as if, at least for phobic wives, that controlled studies support the ideas that the husbands of these wives are struggling with symptoms of their own, that the couple is in a complementary relationship in which the husband is benefiting from the wife's symptoms, and in a significant percentage of the cases, the husbands react negatively to their wives' improvement.

As in the foregoing studies, in the cases that follow, the quid pro quo between the couple concealed the fact that the husband, not the wife, was contending with some major life issue. That issue might have to do with the husband's career, or with a difficulty in adjusting to a life-cycle change. Typically, his struggle involved ambiguity, or an uncertainty as to how to respond to some important question. He could not make up his mind, and so he was indecisive and immobilized regarding the issue at hand. The wife's symptoms served to distract her husband, and allowed him to be defined as the competent one in the relationship. In this sense, the wives were being protective of their husbands, sacrificing their own health in the interest of helping their husbands. The problem is that when everyone, including professionals, is distracted from the husband's problems, his problems never get solved. Although the husband must make up his mind about something, he does not.

The quid pro quo these couples follow not only dictates who will be defined as having the problem, but it also governs how the husband will interact with his wife about her symptoms. If he is patronizing, this becomes a ritualized reaction. If he is exasperated, or demeaning, or is simply ignoring her problems, his way of relating to her becomes stereotyped. The husband's chronic way of relating to his wife around her problems becomes his contribution to maintaining the couple's symptomatic ritual. His part of the overall ritual is also a behavioral communication to his wife. One consequence, therefore, of the husband's always patronizing her, or always becoming exasperated with her, is that his behavior is communicating to her that he does not want the situation to change.

Approaching the wife's symptoms from this point of view has several implications. The obvious implication is that if the wife is having difficulties in helping her husband pull himself together, then to help the wife, the therapist must help the husband. One problem is that the wives typically do not come into therapy with their husbands, they come in alone. The psychiatric community gives them a diagnosis, and usually medication, branding them as the patients and solidifying the unfortunate arrangement the couple already has. When the wife comes in individually, she may be reluctant to implicate her husband because she is protective of him. In the absence of any reason to suspect that the marriage is part of the problem, the professional community can justifiably focus on the wife as the problem. In cases where the wife does complain openly about her husband, some therapists may overreact and push her to leave the marriage. This is a problem if what the wife wants is help *for* her husband, not help with *getting rid of* him.

It could be argued that all of this is just a theory and that therapists are barking up the wrong trees by making assumptions about "underlying" problems. Whether true or not, the idea that the wife's problems are an attempt to protect a struggling husband has several simple and practical ramifications for therapists that cause no harm when taken into consideration.

First, the therapist should be respectful of the husband no matter how much the wife may trash him. A wife may be allowed to be upset with her husband, but for a therapist to reach conclusions about him without meeting him is premature.

Second, it seems reasonable to include a husband in therapy as a helper when the problem is that the wife is totally dysfunctional. Whether or not one assumes the wife's husband has a problem, it seems reasonable to include the husband in the therapy to help the wife over her problems. Again, controlled behavioral therapy studies support the idea of simply including the husband in the wife's treatment. Brownell (1978) found that including husbands in the behavioral treatment for obese women was significantly more effective than individual treatment. These findings replicated earlier studies on including spouses in the treatment of obesity (Mahoney & Mahoney, 1976). Barlow and O'Brien treated two groups of 14 agoraphobic women with behavioral therapy. One group was given individual treatment. In the second group, identical treatment was given in the presence of the women's husbands. Results of the treatment group that included the husbands showed a "substantial" advantage over the individual group. In addition, including the husbands in the treatment resulted in positive changes in social, work, and family functioning that occurred more rapidly than in the individual treatment group (Barlow & O'Brien, 1984).

Finally, whether or not the husband is struggling with some issue, his ritualized, stereotypical way of relating to his wife about her problems is not helping her, and it is usually helpful to her if he can be persuaded to treat her differently. From our point of view, this means pushing the husband to break a rule dictated by the couple's quid pro quo. This is not a minor change to request. Asking a husband who is withdrawn to become more involved in helping his wife with her problems is asking a husband and wife to get closer. This type of directive is not just a minimalistic behavioral directive, but a directive that has bearing on the emotional proximity of the couple, and this is no trivial matter. As the following cases will show, asking for some small, and seemingly reasonable, change in the way the husband is treating his wife's difficulties can result in a monumental struggle of existential proportions.

Including the husband in the wife's therapy means persuading the wife to allow him to come in, recruiting him into the therapy, hearing him out, winning his trust and confidence, and, at a minimum, persuading him to change how he is responding to his wife's symptoms. If the wife is protecting him, many therapists will fail to accomplish the first step. A protective wife must be convinced that her therapist truly wants her husband's help, and is not going to antagonize him. If a protective wife thinks a therapist is anti-male, she is certainly not going to expose her husband to that therapist.

If a therapist gets past a protective wife's reluctance to involve her husband, recruiting her husband into therapy should be done quickly. It is much easier to start a process with all of the principal participants than it is to add someone to a process that has already begun. This means getting the husband in for the first or second appointment. Often a husband will come to the first session if the therapist personally requests that he do so when the initial appointment is set up (Carr, 1998; Heubeck, 1986). If the wife seems reluctant to include him at once, she can come alone the first time, and the husband can attend the second session. It should be assumed that if the wife is reluctant to include her husband in the first session, it is because she wants to scout out the therapist first, before exposing her husband to him or her.

Once a husband attends, to win his trust, the focus must be on the wife's symptoms, not on him or the marriage. This means asking him such questions as: What is your understanding of your wife's problems? Why do you think she is having the problems? What do you think she could do to overcome the problems? How do your wife's problems interfere with your life, or your marriage? What advice does her family (your family, your friends, her friends) have for her or for you to help? What would be different if your wife did not have her problems? What will happen if the problems get worse? Or to the wife: What could your husband do to help? These types of questions focus on the wife's symptoms as the problem being presented to therapy, and so husbands will typically cooperate with answering them. They also begin to reveal how the wife's symptoms are organizing the couple's marriage, and what the husband could do differently to help.

If a husband has been included in this way, and is given tasks to do to help his wife, the therapist is staying within the couple's framework of the wife's being the patient but is simultaneously asking them to change that framework. One implication of the husband's participating in and cooperating with a therapy aimed at helping his wife is that he wants a different marriage. This becomes obvious once it has been established how the wife's symptoms intrude on the marriage.

As will be seen in the following cases, including the husband in the treatment of a severely symptomatic wife does not necessarily mean that he will attend every session. He may end up coming intermittently, or only when a crisis occurs. What is important is how the therapist makes use of the opportunities the husband provides when he does participate.

If a therapist wins the husband's trust and confidence, and succeeds in getting him to relate to his wife's problems in some new manner, it may become obvious that he has some serious difficulties of his own. He may volunteer this information once he trusts the therapist, or it will become apparent through the consequences of asking him to help his wife. Or the wife might see that the therapist is respectful of her husband and volunteer what his conflicts are. Sometimes, after the wife improves, the husband's problems will surface. When, and if, a therapist is presented with struggles the husband is having, attention can be directly focused on helping him. We are not suggesting that in all cases, when a wife improves, or during the course of her therapy, the husband will indicate that he is having difficulty. It has just been our experience, particularly with the most severe cases, that this has proved to be so. When we have succeeded at being helpful, whether the wife's improvement was contingent upon, or just coincidental with, our helping the husband, we do not know. It just appears that often when a wife is presenting severe problems, and the husband is included appropriately, it is discovered that the husband is also having difficulties, and helping him seems to help his wife.

Married with No Children

Rhonda Burnaugh

Cynthia came to her first therapy session alone and in crisis. She was 31 years old, had been married for six years, and had no children. She had a high school education and worked as a cashier in a department store. Shortly after she was married, she had a psychotic episode. She became severely disturbed, stripped nude, and wandered around her neighborhood. At that time, she was diagnosed as having bipolar disorder with psychotic features and put on lithium and Haldol.

In the first session, it was not clear what the crisis was. Cynthia said, "I can't sleep and I think there's something wrong with my medication." As a psychiatric nurse, I work with many clients who are on medication. I hear this statement quite often. Cynthia had been on medication for six years and had been consulting doctors about her symptoms and having her medications adjusted. To accept medication as the total explanation for Cynthia's problems would mean dismissing any other issues in her current situation that might have been contributing to her agitation. Without a thorough exploration of her social situation, it could not properly be assessed whether her complaint was attributable to her medication or to something else. I pushed her to reveal what else might be disturbing her other than medication.

With some reluctance, Cynthia revealed that she had secrets that were upsetting her. She explained that this was her first marriage, but prior to marrying, she had had two "affairs," one with a boyfriend she had known for a while, and one with her sister's boyfriend. Although she said that both had occurred before she was married, she considered them affairs because it was against her religion to have premarital sex. On both occasions, she had become pregnant and had had abortions. She said that, as a Catholic, she was not going to be "forgiven" for her abortions. She felt especially guilty about the "affair" with her sister's boyfriend. She had betrayed her sister. In this first session, Cynthia was rational, and was not psychotic. She said that she was tired of the guilt of having these two secrets and that her husband did not know anything about them.

I explained that the secrets seemed to be a major part of her trouble and asked if she would let me help her with them. I suggested that until we could decide what to do about the secrets, I would be their keeper. Cynthia said she hoped that I could help. She said she did not want to think she would be "mentally ill" for the rest of her life and always have to take medication. The session ended, and as I showed her out of the clinic, we unexpectedly encountered her husband in the waiting room.

The next afternoon, I received a call from a local hospital and was told, "We have Cynthia in the emergency room. We've given her more Haldol. She is extremely psychotic. She said that last night her husband tried to shove his fingers down her throat." Cynthia had been found rummaging through a neighbor's trash cans in search of the family cat. The cat was very old and never to be let outdoors, on strict orders from her husband. He had been given the cat when it was only six weeks old as a birthday gift. Somehow the cat had slipped by her, and now, at 1:00 A.M., the police found her crying and swearing that the cat had been stolen for satanic rituals by vampires. (The police did find the cat the following day. It had been hit by a car and killed.) Cynthia was taken to the hospital and admitted.

Cynthia, a chronic client who had been on medication for six years, was back in the hospital. To become more connected to Cynthia, I decided to visit her there. I did not go to offer therapy, just to visit. A visit is one way to demonstrate that a therapist is taking a more personal interest in a client. My goal was to establish a strong relationship with Cynthia, a relationship I would need if I were going to help.

When I saw Cynthia in the hospital, she was almost catatonic.

She sat on her bed holding her arms stiff and staring blankly ahead. She was almost totally noncommunicative. I talked to her for a little while, and then asked her what had happened between the time I had seen her and when she ended up in the hospital. She had a hard time answering. She could only indicate yes or no. I asked, "Did you get upset when you saw your husband at my office?" She nodded yes. "What upset you about that?" I asked. Finally, she spoke: "He told me that he had secretly wired everything and could hear our entire conversation." Assuming he now knew her secrets, she became psychotic and ended up in the hospital.

I spoke to the psychiatrist who would be in charge of medicating her when she was released. To really help Cynthia, I was going to have to have authority in the case. This would mean two things: (1) I would have to have input regarding her medications. (2) I would have to be in charge of when, and if, she should be hospitalized in the future. If I could help her and her improvement warranted it, I wanted to get her off of the medication and keep her out of the hospital. The psychiatrist agreed to adjust her medications according to how she progressed in treatment. He also agreed not to readmit Cynthia to the hospital without first consulting with me. This was a unique arrangement for a psychiatrist to make with a therapist, but was possible because I had worked closely with this psychiatrist on many cases. He knew me and trusted my judgment. These agreements gave me the authority to carry out the decisions necessary in a serious case like this. In the most difficult cases, we believe it makes sense for the professional most intimately involved with the client to have the most authority.

When Cynthia was discharged, I had a session with her and her husband, Curt. She was convalescing at home after her hospitalization. It turned out that Curt was concerned because Cynthia was in the clinic for her first session with me, when she was supposed to be at work. That was part of their quarrel the night she became psychotic. Although Cynthia was afraid that Curt had overheard her secrets, it was clear that he had not.

When working with clients who are seriously disturbed, difficult choices must be made. The position we work from is to assume that the client is capable of returning to a normal routine and to press the client to return to it as soon as possible. In this approach, if possible, the client is taken off of medication as soon as his or her improvement justifies it. The client is not described as "mentally ill." For Cynthia, this would mean her going back to work and my raising the issue of children with the couple. I took the position with Curt that Cynthia's getting back to her normal routine would help to stabilize her. I asked the couple to set a date for when Cynthia would return to work. They agreed that she should do so in three weeks.

At this point, Cynthia was on large dosages of Haldol and lithium. She was so heavily medicated that she could not conduct herself in a normal manner. If she returned to work in this shape, it was doubtful whether she could function. Even after this latest hospitalization, she continued to question whether she really was ill. She said, "Because I've been in the hospital twice, does that mean I'm sick and I'm always going to have to be on medication?"

Curt insisted that she was very ill. It was important to Curt that Cynthia be labeled the patient. The quid pro quo here was that Cynthia was the patient, and Curt was not. The goal was to get Cynthia out of the patient category without Curt himself becoming a patient. The fact that Cynthia had to take medication branded her as the patient. To pursue the issue of medication, therefore, would be delving into fundamental implicit agreements between the couple.

I took the position that although Cynthia needed the medication at the moment, the hope was that as she improved, the medication would become less necessary. If she did improve, I would advocate that the doctor reduce and, possibly, if her improvement warranted it, eliminate the medication entirely. Curt reluctantly accepted this plan.

After this session, I consulted with the team (Haley, Schiff, and Grove) about the case. Several hypotheses were considered. The fact that Cynthia experienced her first psychotic episode immediately after her marriage suggested that the extended family might have been, and continued to be, involved in an important way.

Often, when symptoms develop immediately after marrying, the person is caught in some way between his or her spouse and one or both sets of parents. Although Curt was controlling, and very paranoid, it is assumed that a husband by himself cannot upset his wife to this magnitude. There must be at least one other person in a power position. It was not clear what either Cynthia's or Curt's relationships were with either set of parents. I assumed, however, that Cynthia's psychosis, and probably her secrets, involved the larger family network.

The fact that the couple had been married for six years and had no children was considered very important. Cynthia's impairment prevented them from having children. After her most recent psychotic episode, Curt told her, "If you can't even take care of a cat, how could you possibly take care of a child?" The couple was stuck at a stage of family life. They were married, but had no children. It was unclear as to whether her psychosis was preventing, or saving, the couple from having children. One consequence of having children is the higher level of commitment to the marriage required. If one or both spouses have doubts about the marriage, or if extended families are opposed to the marriage, the couple will face difficult choices.

We assumed that Cynthia's symptoms were an attempt to help Curt in some way. Although I had no evidence that Curt needed any help, it is assumed in this approach that the symptomatic person is protecting someone and is attempting to help by collapsing. Curt presented himself as strong and competent, but this presentation was happening in a context in which his wife was out of her mind.

The main issue in the case was secrets. It was possible that if the secrets were handled correctly, Cynthia might straighten out. It is our position that it is not a necessary component of a satisfactory marriage for spouses to be completely open. It seems obvious that complete openness between two people is not possible, and would produce a strange relationship if it were. A therapist must decide, based on the case in question, whether or not a particular issue should be brought out into the open. Ordinarily, we do not take the position that a wife should tell her husband about previous abortions. But in this case, we decided that Cynthia should tell Curt her secrets. Having the secrets upset Cynthia enough to land her in the hospital, and made her vulnerable. She was keeping things from her husband, and that gave him power. It gave him power because Cynthia was constantly thinking, "He might know. He might figure this out." Also, it was obvious that Curt suspected that there was some secret. This could make him act suspiciously and distant. Cynthia might then react by being even more concerned that Curt knew or suspected something. Each one's paranoia and suspicions were feeding off of the other's.

Another aspect of the secrets is that they were the basis for the spouses' remaining distant from each other. Cynthia could be obsessed with whether or not Curt knew the secrets, and Curt could be suspicious because Cynthia was behaving oddly. They could use each other's suspicious and paranoid behavior as excuses for why they kept each other at arm's length and why they were not having children. They did not have to face any other potentially threatening issues for why they might be distant. The secrets afforded a way to deal with each other. If the secrets were removed, the spouses either would have to get together, or face what was really keeping them apart. The idea was for Cynthia to put the secrets out on the table and get it over with.

Last, Cynthia believed that she was being punished for having her two abortions by not being allowed to have children. This belief could be viewed as psychotic ideation, or as a guide. Cynthia was linking having or not having children to having or not having secrets. Somehow, these two issues were connected.

The consequences of telling the secrets would have to be examined with Cynthia. One clear possibility was that, if they were revealed, Curt might decide to end the marriage. Cynthia would have to decide whether she was willing to take that risk. An individual session with Cynthia would be set up to discuss how to handle the secrets. The two of us would talk it over at length, but I would take the position that Cynthia should tell the secrets. If she told the secrets, then the couple either could start over or split. The two of us would discuss the possibilities, and if Cynthia decided she wanted to tell the secrets, then a special session with the couple would be scheduled for her to do so.

If Cynthia resisted the idea of telling the secrets, another possibility would be for her not to tell them, but for the couple to make an explicit agreement about secrets. They could jointly decide that whatever happened to either one of them before their marriage was their own personal business and should be allowed to be kept secret. Their own pasts would not be open for discussion. With this approach, at least it would be out in the open between the couple that each was allowed to have secrets about the past.

Cynthia came in alone and we discussed the secrets. I pointed out that it was all right for couples to keep some things private from each other. I explained that different couples make different arrangements regarding secrets. Some reveal everything to each other, and some do not. Some start fresh when they get married. I asked Cynthia if Curt knew how old she was the first time she menstruated and how much she soaked the pad. She said he most certainly did not. I asked her if she had any private fantasies and if Curt knew all of them. She said she did have some very personal fantasies and that Curt did not know them. We agreed that it would be all right for Curt to continue not to know these things. They were Cynthia's business.

The question was whether or not abortions were secrets that should remain her business or whether she should tell Curt about them. We talked about how Curt might react if he knew. She said he might leave her. I agreed that this might happen and that she should really give some thought to whether she wanted to take that risk. I offered her the idea that if she did not want to tell Curt the secrets, she should at least ask that they agree that their pasts were their own business. If Curt agreed, Cynthia's past would become her business. She did not have to feel guilty about keeping secrets about her past. I then explained what my advice would be. I argued that having those secrets got her in the hospital and I thought that for her health's sake she should consider telling him. I said, "Wouldn't it be more sensible to reveal it all to him? Tell him everything and start fresh so that you aren't so vulnerable?"

Cynthia thought her options over and agreed that keeping the secrets disturbed her. She obsessed about Curt's discovering them.

She did not think she could enjoy peace of mind in the marriage while keeping those secrets. She agreed with the idea of telling him. I suggested that she bring Curt to the next appointment so I could help her with confessing to him.

At the next appointment, Cynthia showed up without Curt. She said that she had gone home and told Curt herself. I was skeptical about this, but Cynthia insisted that she had told Curt about the abortions and that he had handled it better than she thought he would. Over the next few weeks, Cynthia proceeded to improve. I decided not to press the secrets issue. Cynthia continued to improve. She went back to work full time and the doctor began to reduce her medication. Eventually, the doctor took her off all of her medication. After she had been back to work for a while, she called and said she did not think she needed to come in anymore. Everything had gone too easily. I was left wondering what would happen next.

Sure enough, Cynthia resurfaced a few months later. She was in crisis and she turned to me. The connection I had established with her paid off. She came in saying she wanted to leave Curt. She said he was abusive. I attempted to get her to describe what abuse he had perpetrated, but she was vague and would not be specific. It was unclear what had prompted her to come in suddenly after several months and say that her husband was abusive and that she wanted out of the marriage. I said, "Let's not be so quick. Let's look at the whole picture. Why don't we talk to Curt? You've been together for more than six years now. Are you sure you want to end it?" Cynthia's thoughts were racing and she was irrational. She was decompensating. I was trying to slow her down. I began to worry and asked her if I could call and talk to Curt. She was strongly against it.

Cynthia continued to deteriorate. I saw her for three days in a row, trying to hold her together and to keep her off medication and out of the hospital. It was a very frustrating situation. Cynthia continued to get worse, but would not allow me to talk to Curt.

Finally, I got her to agree to let me call her mother, who lived in Canada. The situation was desperate. I was hoping to persuade

Cynthia's mother to help. I called her with Cynthia in the office. Her mother was very concerned, but would not come. She said she was "uncomfortable" around Curt. "Uncomfortable" turned out to be a key word. I also called Cynthia's sister in Arizona. Her sister said that if Cynthia would just stay on her medication, her problem would go away. The sister was not going to help either.

As I gleaned more information, the situation was becoming more and more complex. All hell was breaking loose. I was trying to keep the couple together and Cynthia out of the hospital. Then she began hearing voices again. She said she had to be out of the house. She confessed that the secrets she had told me originally were not the real secrets. I asked what the real secrets were. Cynthia confessed that her two "affairs" had taken place after she was married, not before. The first affair occurred soon after she was married. Her sister's child became ill and had to be hospitalized. Cynthia went to help. She ended up sleeping with her sister's husband. I asked if she had told Curt the real secrets. She admitted that she had not. She insisted that she wanted to get out of the house, saying that she was afraid Curt might become violent. Milton Erickson maintained that when a client came to therapy saying that he or she had a secret, whatever secret the client initially told was not the real secret. This turned out to be the case with Cynthia.

What was especially interesting was that Curt's parents brought Cynthia to one of these sessions. She said she felt so awful that she could not drive. She did not trust herself. But she got Curt's parents to drive her. They were waiting in the lobby. I wondered if Cynthia was trying to tell me something. I asked if I could talk to them. Cynthia said No. She then told me that they thought Curt was the perfect son. He was very dutiful and very involved with them.

Cynthia continued to decompensate and I had no place to send her. She finally came in, saying she refused to go home. The question was whether the spouses should separate and if I should encourage it. According to Cynthia, Curt did not know how she felt about the marriage. I could not even get Cynthia to call Curt and let him know she was leaving. I was very frustrated. No matter in which direction I tried to go to include Curt, Cynthia blocked me. I was concerned that Curt might be in bad shape for Cynthia to be so decompensated, but there was nothing I could do.

This was not just Cynthia's maintaining that she was abused and wanted out of her marriage. She was becoming more and more psychotic. An abused wife leaves by going to a shelter. A psychotic wife leaves by going to the hospital. If the couple were going to split, I did not want it ambiguous as to why. Should I call Curt and let him know that his wife was psychotic and needed help? This would be going against Cynthia's insistence that I not call him. It is characteristic of the most difficult cases that therapists invariably will find themselves in situations in which they must decide how much responsibility they should take for their clients and how much responsibility they should allow the clients to have.

Cynthia was insisting that Curt was abusing her, but when I pressed her for details, she offered little information. I asked her, "What is the worst abuse Curt has done?"

Cynthia said, "Once he pushed me down onto the bed. He screams and yells."

"Does he become violent?" I asked.

"No," Cynthia replied.

It did not sound as if Cynthia were in real danger; however, she was adamant about my not talking to Curt. I did not want to take a chance. Cynthia was blocking me from communicating with Curt and I could not help to stabilize her without the assistance of family members. She continued to decompensate. Finally, Cynthia had to be hospitalized. The crisis was over.

Everything was back to square one. While in the hospital, Cynthia did not take responsibility for wanting to separate from Curt. She would not clarify her position concerning the marriage. Instead, she told Curt that I had encouraged her to leave. This was the very thing I was trying to avoid by urging her to let me contact Curt. Curt became very angry with me and organized a meeting in my clinic with Cynthia's psychiatrist and the clinical manager. After all of my efforts, I was on the brink of losing the whole case. I felt completely manipulated by Cynthia. She had pushed me to the limit. Fortunately, I had been in close communication with the psychiatrist throughout the crisis. He had been totally apprised of the situation, and he assured Curt that I was offering the highest quality care. Unfortunately, the only way to appease Curt was for the psychiatrist to agree with Curt that Cynthia was very ill and needed to be back on medication. A total relapse had occurred.

After this meeting, I decided that if I were going to help, I was going to have to take a risk. Without Cynthia's permission, I decided to call Curt and asked to meet with him alone. It is often the case with the most disturbed clients that they do not say what actions they want their therapist to take. The therapist has to figure it out. The problem is that it puts the therapist in a position of having to take responsibility on faith that he or she is doing what the client wants the therapist to do. I decided that Cynthia wanted me to call Curt, but she did not want to take responsibility for his having to come in. She wanted to be able to say to Curt, "I'm not the one who wants you to come in, Rhonda is." I had to go through hell to figure this out.

Curt did come in. I appeased him by saying, "You are right, Cynthia is very sick at the moment. That is very apparent. For me to help her, I have to have your help. You live with her. You see her every day, I do not. You are in the best position to help her. For me to help, you must be willing to let me know what is going on. Otherwise, what just happened with Cynthia could happen again." Curt agreed that Cynthia would have to go back to work, and do all of the things she had done before in order to get back on her feet. If she improved as before, however, this time Curt was to call me at the first sign of trouble. Curt would come in with Cynthia. In the previous crisis, I had not been connected enough to Curt to get a change. I was anticipating another go-around with Cynthia, but this time I wanted to be in a position to involve Curt.

Soon after this meeting, Cynthia went back to work and made steady progress. Things were quiet for months. Then, as predicted, Cynthia called and requested an appointment. I asked for Curt to come, but she came alone.

She again brought up the fact that she was tormented by guilt over the secrets. We spoke about what a couple with their backgrounds would ordinarily be doing at this point in their marriage. A couple in their early 30s, with their backgrounds and married for six years, most likely would have had, or be having, or at least be planning to have children. Cynthia spontaneously said, "Curt won't have children with me. He says I'm too sick." She also explained that she herself was uncomfortable with the idea of having children with Curt when she was keeping such big secrets from him.

Two things were now clear. First, when Cynthia was competent and not defined as a mental patient (in this case, meaning she was acting normally and was also off medication), the question of having a child was on the table. Her condition could not be used as an excuse for not having children. But having children required Cynthia to be honest with Curt about the secrets. If Cynthia were going to be as committed to Curt as having children would require, they would first have to resolve the matter of the secrets. When the couple reached this point in the cycle, the secrets would not be brought out into the open. Cynthia would then relapse, removing the pressure to tell the secrets and deal with the question of having children. Once she relapsed, secrets became the babbling of a crazy person and children were out of the question.

Second, it looked as if three possibilities existed for Cynthia: (1) She could tell the secrets, and she and Curt would work it out and go on and have children. (2) She would tell the secrets, which would upset Curt, and he would want a divorce. (3) Cynthia would not tell the secrets, would remain labeled a patient, and would have periodic relapses to ensure the impossibility of either having children or splitting. The idea that Cynthia could tell the secrets and the couple would stay married and not have children did not seem likely. They both obviously hoped to have children eventually.

I explained these three possibilities to Cynthia. I said, "You are at a point in your life where you have to make some decisions. You can remain the same, keep the secrets, and continue to go in and out of the hospital. You can do that and have a marriage that is emotionally distant. Or you can decide that you and Curt will not have secrets and go on and have children. But that possibility requires a risk. You have to tell the secrets. You might end up divorced." I asked her to go home and to think it over. If she decided to tell the secrets, we would set up a meeting and she could tell Curt in my office. She was not to tell him at home. I wanted to avoid what she had done the last time, when she lied to me about telling Curt, when really she had not. To block her from trying this again, I counted on her being protective of Curt. I said, "If you decide to tell him, he will need support hearing them. It is only fair that you bring him here so I can help him with it."

One week later, Cynthia came in with Curt to tell the secrets, nine months and one hospitalization after I had first proposed that she tell him. It was like giving birth. We got together at 9:00 A.M., with Curt's having to go directly to work after the session. I tried to make it easy for them. I started by asking Curt what he knew and what he had guessed about Cynthia's past. I was hoping that he would bring up the secrets himself. Cynthia would then just have to confirm his suspicions. He said he thought there was something she did not want to tell him, but he did not know what it was.

Cynthia volunteered that she had had an affair after she and Curt were married. Curt listened and sat quietly for a moment. Then he said, "Is that all that this has been about? I had an idea in the back of my head that you had done that." Curt was not surprised. He had suspected all along. Curt said he forgave her and spontaneously got out of his chair and hugged Cynthia. He was kind and supportive. He said, "Now we can go on from here." Cynthia cried. It looked pretty good so far.

Then Curt asked, "Is that the only secret?" When Cynthia became nervous, she acted like a little girl. When Curt asked his question, she got a little girl's look on her face. She looked down at the floor, and then over at me. I knew there was one more secret. Finally, Cynthia said, "Yes. That is the only secret." Curt looked suspicious but accepted her answer. He then got up and said he had to go to work.

It often happens in family therapy that, in a flash of seconds, a family will act out its pattern in front of a therapist. This little scene of Curt's asking Cynthia, Cynthia's getting a childish look on her face suggesting one thing, but then saying another, had been played out countless times. The last part of this pattern was the most important. Cynthia nonverbally indicated one thing, but then said another. Curt did not press the issue. Explicitly, he accepted her verbal statement, but he did so with a suspicious look, implying he did not believe her. This sequence was a portrait of their marriage. Cynthia would lie and Curt would not press the issue.

It is characteristic of family members of a severely disturbed client that they hesitate with the client at a crucial moment. The hesitant person is often in a position of power over the client, like a parent of a psychotic youth who hesitates to insist on normal behavior just at the moment when such insistence would have the most impact. When needed, the powerful person does not assert himself or herself. Often it is a male who is not asserting himself. In this case, the man not asserting himself was a husband, not a parent.

The couple had acted out their usual pattern in my presence. If allowed to go on, they would just be repeating their cycle. Nothing would change. I had a critical decision to make, and I had only a few seconds to make it. Cynthia lied. Curt knew it, but did not press her.

I looked at Cynthia and said, "You know that was not the only secret."

"I know. I have to tell him," Cynthia replied.

We ran after Curt and found him in his car in the parking lot. I said, "Cynthia still has something to say to you."

Curt looked at Cynthia and said, "Let's have it."

Cynthia told about the second affair, the one with her sister's husband. Curt stared angrily. "All right. Get in the car and let's get out of here," he barked. Cynthia got into the car and they drove away.

For three agonizing hours, I waited. Finally, a call came. It was Curt. He said, "I have thought about this and I have decided that Cynthia and I are through. For six years, her whole family has considered me an asshole. None of them would ever visit. Now I find out that Cynthia slept with her sister's husband, and her entire side of the family knew! They knew, but they considered me the ass! The whole marriage has been a charade. I cannot ever have children with this woman." Curt mentioned their not having children spontaneously. Having children and having secrets were definitely tied together. Cynthia's mother's statement that she was "uncomfortable" around Curt now had new meaning. It was now clear how the secrets involved the larger family. The discomfort came from knowing the secrets. Everyone knew but Curt!

In this case, we focused on one issue, one set of behaviors, Cynthia's telling or not telling secrets. Contained in that one issue was how the couple related to each other with distance and suspicions; boundaries around Cynthia and her family that excluded Curt; major life decisions, such as having children; a struggle of Curt's not asserting himself; and Cynthia's attempting to arrange for him to do so; and probably much more than we could ever speculate about. We assume that symptomatic behavior is always laden with multiple meanings. By focusing on one problem, in this case the secrets, we were simultaneously touching on a multitude of issues. As Minuchin has pointed out, "The past is contained in the present" (Minuchin & Nichols, 1993).

My conversation with Curt ended with his volunteering that he was not just going to abandon Cynthia. He would help her to get organized and move, but the marriage was over. Two weeks later, Curt drove Cynthia to her mother's home. The split-up was consensual. Cynthia handled it with no psychotic symptoms of any kind.

Two months later, I called Cynthia to check on her. She was still at her mother's. She was planning to go back to school. She and Curt were struggling with the normal things couples struggle with in a divorce. The divorce was proceeding. Cynthia was in very good spirits. Despite the fact that the couple was splitting up, Cynthia said she felt better than she had in a long time. She said that getting the secrets out made her feel as though a huge weight had been lifted from her shoulders.

I followed up again six months later. Cynthia was still at her mother's home but was in college. Her divorce was final. She had been totally off of her medication for over 11 months, had been through the breakup of her marriage, and had had no psychotic symptoms.

Discussion

Although there were times during the case in which the situation was totally confusing, after the secrets were told and the case played out, everything made sense. Cynthia's entire family was in a coalition with her against Curt by keeping the secrets from him. On the other hand, Curt's parents had placed him on a pedestal. He was a very dutiful son. He lived close to his parents. He was an only child. He often visited them and helped them do things. He had a very important role in his family. To stay with Cynthia after the secrets were out would have meant a real fall from that pedestal. The parents would not have been pleased that the perfect son's wife was unfaithful. They were willing to tolerate a crazy wife, but not an unfaithful one. Curt's family's needs were the priority and precluded him from committing himself to Cynthia in the way that having a child would have required. The way Curt said, "I'm not going to have children with you now," sounded as though he had not planned to in any event.

The problem was that Cynthia's "illness" was the pretense for why. Instead of acknowledging that Cynthia had secrets that tormented her, she was defined as sick and had to function below her potential. She was working as a maid, but she came from a college-educated family.

When Cynthia improved, it appeared as though she wanted Curt to prevail upon her to tell the secrets, and he never did. She would then relapse and suffer the consequences of having them. Finally, Cynthia had to be the one to tell the secrets, without Curt's insisting on it. The act of her telling and accepting the consequences cleared up her psychosis. Pretending no longer was required, and Cynthia had had to do a lot of pretending. She had to pretend with Curt. She had to pretend with his parents. She put her whole family in a situation in which they had to pretend.

One characteristic of psychosis is that the symptoms allow the client to escape taking a position on anything. We assume that the psychotic client is in a social context that demands that he or she avoid defining his or her relationships with others (Haley, 1959). Cynthia's having the secrets allowed both her and Curt to stay at arm's length and created an ambiguous situation. Instead of committing themselves to each other and having children, or not having children and splitting, they both avoided clarifying their respective positions by hiding behind Cynthia's "illness."

In addition, since Cynthia's family knew the secrets, Cynthia could not tell the secrets voluntarily without being disloyal to her family of origin. She was trapped in a situation in which keeping the secrets made her ill, and telling them made her disloyal.

A solution for Cynthia would be for her to arrange to have someone make her tell. The obvious first choice would have been Curt. She did extreme things to force Curt to take charge. Cynthia was trying to get Curt to press her to tell. If Curt had done so, such an act would have said, "Let's wipe the slate clean and start over." It would have committed him more to her and less to his family. It would also have gotten Cynthia off the hook with her family. She could tell them she told because Curt made her tell.

Curt's not insisting that she reveal the secrets, however, was communicating his ambivalence about the marriage. It suggested that he preferred to keep himself distant from Cynthia. Her dilemma was that if she initiated telling the secrets, that would not have been Curt's clarifying *his* position. He would have escaped having to take responsibility for what he wanted.

Thinking of the problem in this way, their breakup was a result of her being the one who finally had to tell. If he had made her tell, that would have put him in a better position. He could have told his parents, "I made her tell." But the way it happened, he could not save face, and he had to leave her.

It took courage to push Cynthia to tell the secrets. She put the therapist in a position of having to take responsibility for a major issue. In the absence of Curt's insisting, the therapist decided to. What Cynthia got the therapist to do was what she wanted her husband to do: be bold enough apparently to transgress her expressed wishes and take a stand; to be visible.

A First Child

Janet was a 30-year-old woman, married, with one child, an 18-month-old girl. She and her husband, Daniel, were both professionals. At my request, they both came to the first interview. Janet was of medium height and very underweight. She walked hunched over, shuffling her feet as if she were 90 years old. Although very affluent, Janet was wearing sweat pants and no makeup. She looked terrible.

Janet was convinced that her cervix was gradually disintegrating. She felt this. She was also convinced that her uterus was floating around inside of her, and that her spine was descending, putting pressure on her pelvic bone. She experienced a constant dull pressure above her pelvic region.

Janet had these sensations continuously. She could not work. She was very weak. The psychiatrist who referred her to me was at a loss. There were no medications he could offer that helped. He was very worried that she was going to die because she took such terrible care of herself. She was just withering away. Every morning she dragged herself up out of bed. It took all her effort to get from the bed to the shower. Sometimes, she could wash and dress by herself, sometimes she needed Daniel to help.

Janet had been to the Cleveland Clinic, but the doctors there could find nothing wrong. She had been extensively evaluated at three hospitals in Columbus, Ohio. Nothing physically wrong was found. She had a list of six or seven physicians of various specialties who had examined her and had found nothing. She had been in therapy for the past 14 months with a therapist who was confronting her about her "delusions." Eventually, Janet fired the therapist and found her way to me.

During the month preceding her first appointment with me, she had made two suicide attempts. In her last suicide attempt, two weeks prior to my first interview, she overdosed on sleeping pills. She said she got up that morning and could not put her shirt on. She just gave up. She reported that although she did not have a specific plan to harm herself, she had suicidal feelings every day.

There were major consequences to Janet's symptoms. First, Janet could not care for her baby. She was too weak. During the week, her mother-in-law came in to take care of the child. On the weekends, Daniel took over. Another consequence of her symptoms was that Daniel was now working out of the home. He had an office elsewhere, but he moved his work to their home because Janet was incapable of doing anything. Considering her social class and ethnic background, Janet was in a totally abnormal situation. She was not working, although she had a professional degree. Daniel worked at home, so the partners were together 24 hours a day. Janet's mother-in-law came to the house and took care of Janet's baby, while Janet was distant from the child.

I asked Janet what she would be doing if she were better that she could not do now. The first thing she said was, "I'd hold my baby. I'd change my baby's diapers. I'd feed my baby." She said she would also go back to work full-time, and have a nanny take care of the baby during the day.

I asked Daniel, "Do you think she ever exaggerates this pain?"

He said, "I don't think she exaggerates, I think it's a total fabrication! When I check on her she is just sitting in the chair watching television like nothing's wrong with her." He said this in front of her.

Janet became very angry because Daniel did not believe her. She was convinced that she had a physical problem and was determined to discover what it was. Daniel said that five to ten times a day, Janet would stand in front of the mirror, take her clothes off, and examine herself to see whether her spine had collapsed anymore in the last hour. She insisted she could see it. He could not see anything abnormal. Janet had been convinced she had something medically wrong with her since shortly after the birth of the baby, when her bizarre symptoms began.

Janet had a father and a sister who lived in another state. Her mother was deceased. She said, "I didn't want my child to have a family like mine. My family was totally mother dominated." I asked her what she meant by that. She said, "My father wasn't involved with us kids. I wanted a balance where I would be involved with my child, and my husband would be also." I asked if she thought Daniel was a good father and involved sufficiently with their child. Janet said he was. He had to be.

Daniel's mother lived in town and was on her own. His father was deceased and he had a grandmother who lived in a nursing home. Daniel also had a younger sister and a younger brother, both of whom lived far away. At the first interview, Daniel explained that he and his mother were at odds with each other over the care of his grandmother, but I did not get the details about this until later. At one point after Janet had developed all of her problems, Daniel's mother told her, "Your problems are ruining my son." Janet, on the other hand, complained that Daniel spent too much time dealing with his mother.

I asked them both what would happen if the problem were to get worse. They both said that Janet would have to go to an institution. They would put her in a nursing home at age 30! Daniel then said he wanted her hospitalized immediately. He was already prepared to have her institutionalized! Somehow I had to block this. To institutionalize her now would only make change less likely. I told them I had great doubts that she would get over this problem without being in her natural environment. I said, "If you're worried that she's suicidal, I don't want you to take any chances. The hospital can protect her for a few days, and get her past a suicidal period, but it isn't going to get her over these difficulties." I asked Daniel to keep a close eye on Janet. I said, "If she becomes suicidal again, either you or a hospital must monitor her until she feels better."

Soon after this first interview, Janet began to complain more about her spine and her activity level deteriorated further. My thought was that she got worse because Daniel had accused her of fabricating her symptoms. She had to prove that something was really wrong. Janet was so angry with Daniel for not believing her about her symptoms that I had to help her improve without its proving that Daniel was right about her not having a medical problem. I had to help Janet save face.

My initial hypothesis about the problem was that the couple was struggling to adjust to the birth of the baby. Janet's symptoms were in relation to the consequences of their having their first child. This hypothesis was based on the fact that the symptoms began shortly after the birth of the baby, and on Janet's own response to the question of what she would do if she were better. The first thing she said was that she would take care of her baby. I was wondering if Daniel was struggling to adjust to having the baby. Janet's symptoms were her attempt to help him. Faced with her problems, he had to pull himself together and focus on the family.

To intensify my relationship with Janet, I spoke privately to her about her body image. Erickson had developed a therapeutic procedure that focused on body image (Haley, 1973). The therapist instructs the client to, while at home and in private, strip nude, and examine himself or herself in front of a full-length mirror. The client is asked to really look at himself or herself, and to be as fair as possible in assessing what the client feels are his or her best features, and to report the findings to the therapist. This was a very appropriate idea for this client, because she was already examining her nude body in front of her mirror. But this particular directive was meant to help intensify my therapeutic relationship with her. It would be asking her to do a very intimate and personal thing. The idea was that if she completed this task, it would connect her to me in a more powerful way.

Janet's deterioration after the first session made one thing clear. Whatever I came up with would have to include some sort of physical intervention to help her over what she insisted was a physical complaint. To gain her cooperation, I was going to have to offer an intervention that would allow her to maintain the view that her problem was medical. I could ask her to go on a special diet, or to adhere to an exercise program or to some new-age medical procedure. Before proposing anything like this to her, I would have to consult her primary physician and get the physician's approval. That way, whatever I offered would carry the weight of the medical establishment.

Given the number of doctors on Janet's case, and her obsession, it was imperative that I connect with her doctors. Their way of handling Janet could be part of the problem. With so many doctors, it was possible that Janet was being triangulated between two of them. If the doctors disagreed over how to treat her, she would be receiving conflicting advice, and this could be contributing to her problems. It was also important to understand how the doctors interacted with her. They might be patronizing her by listening to her complaints, and just dismissing her. Or they might be insisting there was nothing wrong with her, spurring her on to find a physiological basis for her symptoms. In either case, if the way the doctors were approaching her was upsetting to her, she could be punishing them by continuing to go to them with her problems (Haley, 1996). Obviously, there was more contributing to her symptoms than just how the doctors were dealing with her. With the doctors so involved, however, it was very important that I include their treatment in my analysis of her social situation, and decide if I needed to intervene with them.

One assumption in Strategic Therapy is that normal behavior produces normal thoughts, cognition, and emotional states (Haley, 1997). Janet was in a very abnormal social context and I was assuming that this was greatly exacerbating her symptoms. It was obvious that I had to get her more connected to her baby. I was very concerned about her mother-in-law's coming over to take care of the child. Having her mother-in-law take care of the child while Janet was present was a very abnormal setup. Her mother-in-law was the same woman who complained that Janet was "ruining my son." Also, given the conflict between Daniel and his mother, having his mother take care of his baby on a daily basis did not seem advisable. I needed a plan that would move the mother-in-law out and Janet closer to the baby.

The main question I had initially was: What should my unit for therapy be? Therapists must always decide on their unit. Will they work with the client individually? If the client is married, will they include the spouse? Will the therapy focus on the family at home? Will it focus on extended family? Family Therapy has called attention to this issue, and depending on the therapist's theoretical orientation, any of the above could be pursued. In our approach, we do not have a rigid rule about which unit to choose. It is our view that therapists must be skilled at working with any possible unit, and must decide on the unit on which they will focus, given the particular case and problem at hand. In this way, the therapist has options and must choose the option that seems to present the most expedient way to resolve the client's problems.

In this particular case, selecting the unit was a difficult decision. On the one hand, Janet was furious at Daniel for not taking her problems seriously, and was willing to go to great lengths to prove to him that her problems were medical. This suggested that the "cure" might have to involve punishing Daniel for his attitude. He might have to take a week off to help her. He might have to purchase camping equipment, and take his wife into the country to take advantage of the curative benefits of the great outdoors. Janet's anger at Daniel suggested that she might cooperate with an intervention that would seriously inconvenience him. Also, if he were in fact struggling with issues related to their having a baby, I would have to help him in some way. By thinking in this manner, it made sense to include him in the unit for therapy.

One issue was making it difficult to decide how to include him, however. Janet had made two suicide attempts in the past month. She felt suicidal on a daily basis. It was not clear how Daniel was related to this. It could be that Janet wanted him more involved with her, taking her problems more seriously. Her suicide attempts could be acts designed to get closer to him. Or it could be that she felt trapped with him and her symptoms were an attempt to get distance from him. When suicide is a concern, it is often wise not to push a suicidal spouse closer to, or farther apart, from the other spouse, unless the therapist understands what the suicidal client wants. After one interview, I was not sure what Janet wanted in relation to Daniel. She said she wanted to be closer to her child. She did not mention her husband. I decided that until I understood the situation better, I would start by working primarily with Janet alone, and include Daniel periodically. Once I understood the situation more fully, I would include Daniel more often.

At our second appointment, I started with Janet alone. I asked if she was agreeable to setting a goal of getting more involved with her baby. She agreed, but said that her condition limited her greatly. I suggested that she and her husband bring their child to the next session so I could observe what she could and could not do with her.

I asked her what she wanted from Daniel. She said she was not sure what she wanted from him. She said he was conducting himself so badly regarding her difficulties that she was very angry with him. She also said that he frightened her. I asked her to explain, and she told me about the situation between Daniel and his mother. Daniel's grandmother was in ill health, and had been placed in what Daniel considered a substandard nursing home. He wanted her in a better facility, but his mother did not. He and his mother were locked in a bitter battle over this. At one point, Daniel was so upset with his mother that he attempted to take legal action against her. Janet was taken aback by this. If he were capable of acting this way to his own mother, what might he do to her? She had spent most of her time with her previous therapist complaining about Daniel, and the previous therapist urged her to leave him. Janet was very uncertain as to what she wanted to do. She was in no condition to go anywhere, and her first choice was to salvage her family. She wanted Daniel to change, but she was close to giving up on him.

It was not clear whether Janet wanted closeness to or distance from Daniel. I needed an approach that would cover both possibilities. The approach I would offer would require Janet to improve no matter what she wanted. I explained that, on the one hand, if she wanted to save her marriage, her condition would have to improve. Daniel did not have an unlimited tolerance for her problems, and sooner or later, he would get fed up if she did not improve. She agreed. On the other hand, if she decided to leave him, she was certainly not in any shape to do so. If she wanted out, she had to improve. Either way, she had to get better. It was clear that my taking a position on her marriage would have been an error. Although she was unhappy with her previous therapist for pushing her to leave Daniel, if I pushed her to stay with her husband, she would feel that I did not appreciate how upsetting he was to her. This plan allowed her to improve whether she wanted to be closer to or farther apart from Daniel.

I inquired about her doctors. She said that she had one primary-care physician who was coordinating her care, and referring her to various specialists. She gave me permission to speak to her primary-care physician. I explained that before she and I considered what she might do to improve, I first needed to consult her doctors. As obsessed as she was with her physical condition, it would have been premature for me to offer any ideas on how she might improve without first talking to the doctors.

Next, I brought in Daniel. I explained that I would be starting out by working primarily with Janet individually, but that I would need his periodic participation regarding specific issues. I then asked him about the situation concerning him and his mother. He said essentially what Janet had reported. Since his mother was in the house every day, I asked him if this conflict might not be creating an awkward situation for everyone. He said it was.

Both Janet and Daniel were professionals. When I asked what their plan for child care was prior to Janet's becoming ill, they said that they had planned to hire a nanny. I asked them why they could not do that now. This thought had never occurred to them. I asked the two of them to talk this over, and to discuss it with Daniel's mother. I stressed to Daniel that despite Janet's limitations, I thought it would help her improve if she could be more involved with the baby. He agreed. He was very concerned about how detached Janet was from their child. I explained that to get her more involved with the child, we would need his mother's help as she was currently the child's primary caretaker. Privately, I was thinking of a strategy to involve the mother-in-law in a positive way. I wanted to move her out of the child-care role, but I did not want the couple just to summarily expel her. The session ended with my asking them to return next time with their child and Daniel's mother.

Before my next session, I had a long talk with Janet's doctor. The doctor was clearly exasperated with Janet, and was totally convinced that there was absolutely nothing medically wrong with her. Janet had seen every imaginable specialist, and had had countless tests, all turning up nothing. The way the doctor spoke made me concerned that she was alienating Janet. I told her that after Janet had gone so far with insisting that something was physically wrong with her, she was not going to drop it now. We had to help her find a face-saving way out of this. I was politely suggesting that she treat Janet more respectfully. I explained that I was thinking about suggesting a plan to Janet that would include something physical, such as a special diet, or an exercise program that would allow her to improve, and give credit to the physical interventions. That way, she would not have to admit the problems might be psychological. The doctor liked this idea, and agreed to make referrals to both a homeopath and an exercise physiologist. We also agreed to keep in regular contact.

Janet, her husband, her child, and her mother-in-law came to the third session. The baby was very well mannered. She played on the floor while the grownups talked. Since our last appointment, the three adults had discussed the idea of hiring a nanny to take care of the child to relieve the grandmother of this duty. I explained that I thought it would help Janet immensely if she could do as much as she was physically able to do with the child. The grandmother approved. I asked Janet to spend some time in the session playing with the child. All she could do was sit on her chair and talk to the baby. Janet was too limited physically, and the baby was too active for her to handle alone. It was very sad. Her child was responsive to her, but she said she was not able to get on the floor and play with her.

I proposed to everyone that we set a goal of getting Janet more involved with the baby before a nanny was hired. I wanted the grandmother and Janet to get together in a positive way before the grandmother was dismissed from her caretaking duties. The grandmother said she would be glad to help, and volunteered that Janet could play with the child at home on Janet's bed, with the grandmother present in case Janet needed help. Janet really liked this idea. I asked the two women if they could structure some time every day for Janet to play with the baby. Once a routine of Janet and the baby playing together had been established, the couple could hire a nanny, and the grandmother could leave, knowing she had helped Janet become more involved with the child. Everyone liked this plan.

My next session was with Janet individually. In this session, I would set up my strategy. I told her that her doctor and I had had a long talk, and that we would like to propose a new strategy for how she might improve. I pointed out that the medical establishment continued to be mystified by her illness, and that traditional medical techniques might not ever be capable of uncovering her problem, or helping her improve. Thus, the doctor and I were suggesting that she take a more holistic approach. The doctor wanted to refer her to a homeopath for some suggestions on diet and life-style changes, and possibly to an exercise physiologist. Janet loved this. I was accepting the framework of her having a physical problem. None of the other professionals had done this. I was concerned, however, that it might be difficult for Janet to commit herself to any plan that was proposed in the absence of a definitive medical diagnosis. She admitted that she wanted desperately to know what was really wrong with her. I replied that I was concerned that she might never know, and that she had to improve regardless. She agreed with this.

By the next session, she had set up her first appointment with a homeopath. She came in looking somewhat better. She walked more freely, and did not act as though she were in constant pain. She reported that she did stand in front of her mirror nude, and that she could not find anything attractive about herself. She said that she once was very satisfied with her appearance, but had deteriorated so badly that she could barely look at herself. I thought this was a good sign. She once felt she was attractive, and maybe the goal of becoming more attractive again would be another motivator for her to take better care of herself. The body-image intervention had multiple effects. It had an unexpected effect on her obsessively removing her clothes and checking in a mirror several times a day to see if her spine had changed. It was one more thing that made Daniel view her as crazy. After my request for her to examine herself, she stopped standing in front of the mirror naked. The directive had a paradoxical effect. Most important, this was a very personal thing for a male therapist to ask of a female client. For her to report in detail to me about something as intimate as her view of her own body made her more connected to me. It gave me more influence with her. As the therapy progressed, I would need every ounce of this influence.

She also reported that she and her mother-in-law had begun

their plan of structuring time for Janet to play with the baby, and she found she could do more with the child than she originally thought. In less than a month, the couple had hired a nanny, and the mother-in-law no longer was in charge of the child. This was a huge change. Janet spent more and more time with the child, and eventually began to take her out to the park to play. After Janet began to be more active with her child, she stopped reporting that she had any suicidal feelings. Although her functioning would improve and relapse during the course of therapy, she never became suicidal again. The grandmother remained involved by coming over once in a while to visit the baby. She was now acting like a grandmother, not like the child's mother.

Just after the nanny was hired, I made a home visit. What I observed was incredible. The house was a very expensive home in an elite suburb. But inside, it was completely trashed. It was a total disaster. Daniel's papers were piled everywhere. It is striking how often a messy house goes with the messiest cases. Janet was very displeased with the mess and embarrassed for me to see it. I met with Janet in her living room. She shuffled around the house as if barely capable of getting herself from one room to the next. While she struggled to move about, Daniel was busy with work. Janet acted as though she could die at any moment, and Daniel just went about his business as if nothing was wrong with her. Finally, Daniel did join us. For the nine thousandth time, the couple got into a fight about whether or not there was really something wrong with Janet. The visit gave me a clear picture of the couple's symptomatic rituals. I suppose I already knew what was going on between them, but actually seeing it made it graphic. Janet was exaggerating and Daniel was minimizing, and they were both willing to fight to the death to prove their points.

Janet did get connected with a homeopathic doctor, who made several suggestions. Exercise was one of them. She referred her to an exercise physiologist, who put her on a daily program. Janet began taking better care of herself, and it showed in her appearance and in her walk. Her shuffle had reduced dramatically. She even got to the point of going to work one or two days a week. She began to complain more about her husband than about her symptoms.

Now that Janet's suicidal feelings had subsided, I decided to include Daniel more in the sessions. I attempted a straightforward approach of trying to help the couple negotiate the issues on which they disagreed. Janet wanted Daniel to clean up his mess in the house, and not to pressure her for sex. They were having sex regularly, despite Janet's complaints that it was physically painful. It was one more way in which they fought about whether or not Janet had a medical problem.

After a few sessions of focusing on marital issues, Janet relapsed. Although she remained involved with her baby, she stopped going to work, reduced her overall activities, and went back to constant complaining about her symptoms. It was clear after this relapse that to solve the problem, I was going to have to change my approach. Janet's relapse was in relation to her husband. The main aspect of Janet's problems focused on the intense struggle she and Daniel were engaged in with each other. They were both stubborn and unyielding. The battle was being fought over whether or not Janet really had anything physically wrong with her, and the consequences for their marriage if she did. This fight absorbed both of them. I wondered to myself what the consequences would be for their marriage if Janet were *well*.

After having seen Janet individually, I was concerned that Daniel might have felt I was biased when the therapy turned to focusing on issues between the spouses. I was not connected enough to Daniel. I decided to shift gears and work more with Daniel. I would continue with Janet and even bring the two together occasionally, but my emphasis would be on Daniel. My attention would be on what changes Daniel wanted. What would make him happy? What would he like to be different? The idea was that if he were happier, Janet might improve. The assumption was that her symptoms were protective of him. They organized him. If he had problems, he had to put them aside to focus on her. If this assumption were true, then solving his problems would reduce the need for Janet to be symptomatic. One clear problem was the ongoing argument between Daniel and his mother. Janet had even stated in the first interview that he devoted too much of his energy to fighting with his mother. Clearly, attention could be devoted to this issue.

One additional thing was becoming clear. Improvement would be hard to judge in this case. Janet attended every session and complained about her symptoms. If allowed, she would complain about her back for the entire session, or some other bizarre sensation. If something changed that she wanted, she was not going to drop her complaints because this would imply that her symptoms were due to whatever had just changed, and not to a medical condition. She had gone to such great lengths with insisting that she had a medical problem that at best she was only going to reduce her complaining gradually. Using the intensity of her complaints as a barometer for improvement would make it difficult to understand what changes she wanted, and whether they were occurring. Instead, her actual functioning would have to be used as a yardstick. Did she go back to work? Did she interact with the baby? Did she take better care of herself? Changes in these areas would have to be used to measure success.

I spoke to Janet about the idea of my helping Daniel. She loved it. She was very worried about him and wanted him to get help. Her response was evidence that the assumption that her problems were protective of him was correct.

After proposing this to Janet, I saw Daniel individually. I explained to him that I was worried about him. He had a wife who was falling apart and doing nothing. He had a grandmother whose health was deteriorating but was not receiving the care that he would like to see her receive. And he had a mother with whom he was fighting bitterly about it. I said I thought Janet might do better if he had a better situation. He downplayed his problems, and said he was a very strong person and had made up his mind to endure what life delivered. The way in which he responded suggested he had resigned himself to his predicament. He was not considering how he might assert himself to produce changes.

I asked him what he would change if he could organize his situation in any way he wanted. The first thing he mentioned was getting his grandmother into a better facility. However, his mother did not want to pay the extra cost. He also said that if he were not so restricted by his wife's problems, he would work outside the home and devote more time to his work. I asked him if he would indulge me and let me try to assist with some of these matters. He agreed.

Daniel and I looked at the disagreement between him and his mother. He was very angry with her for not providing what he felt his grandmother needed. I asked if some sort of compromise were possible.

"What would that be?" he asked.

I asked him whether, if he were willing to pay the difference in cost for a better facility, his mother might not be willing to move his grandmother. She could continue to pay the same amount she was paying now, but his grandmother would be receiving superior care. He and his mother could shop around together to find a new facility. He liked this idea and said his mother just might go for it. His mother agreed, and they eventually moved the grandmother into a more expensive facility for which Daniel helped to pay. This was a big change that Janet said she was happy to see. Daniel's entire family had been struggling over this issue, and she was sick of the tension it created.

The question of Daniel's wanting to spend more time with work proved to be more complicated. After my home visit, it was clear to me that there were two major problems: (1) Daniel worked out of the home, forcing the couple to be together 24 hours a day, seven days a week. They were driving each other crazy. (2) The house was a disaster, mostly because Daniel's papers were scattered all over. I began to realize what a change it would be if Daniel were to go back to working at his office. The house would get cleaned up, something Janet wanted, and the spouses would have time apart from each other. It would be so different if Daniel would leave at 8:00 in the morning and not return until 5:00 P.M. I proposed this to Janet, and she loved the idea. But Daniel did not. He was very reluctant to go back to working at his office and it was not clear why, especially in light of his desire to work more. His stated reason was that he needed to be home for the baby, although they had already hired a nanny.

During this period, Janet's father came to visit from California to be supportive of Janet. This meant a lot to her. She felt outnumbered by Daniel and his family. While her father was visiting, I invited him to a session. He turned out to be a very nice man who was very concerned about his daughter. I spoke with him in private and asked what he thought would help Janet. He said he was appalled by the condition of the house, and that when Janet was growing up, she had not been accustomed to such conditions. I explained that I had been trying to persuade Daniel to go back to working out of his office, which would result in most of the mess getting cleaned up. He thought it was a very good idea, and told me that if I could get Daniel to do it, I would be worth twice whatever fee I was charging. He characterized Daniel as a very stubborn man. I asked him if he would be willing to help me try to persuade Daniel.

I brought Daniel in and Janet's father and I spoke with him about his going back to working out of his office. Janet's father very diplomatically explained why he felt it would help Janet improve. He was obviously awkward at asserting his views, not wanting to interfere with what he said was the couple's business. Daniel listened and agreed to the idea. The trouble was that he had agreed before, but had not done anything about it. I thought that if he made the promise in front of Janet's father, he might go through with it. But again, Daniel did not follow through.

I was beginning to realize that Daniel was not changing anything related to marital issues or the way he interacted with Janet. No matter what approach I used, he would not cooperate. Obviously, there was something important I did not understand.

Soon after this, Janet told me that she and Daniel had the best relationship before the birth of their child. I asked what was different then. She said that they went their own ways and were very independent of each other. The situation was now becoming clear. Janet was happiest when the two lived independently. Before their child was born, they were essentially living parallel lives. Although Janet was saying she preferred such an arrangement, it was not clear that Daniel wanted that kind of marriage.

The problem was that living parallel lives might be possible for two people, but becomes much more difficult when a baby is introduced into the picture. In the first session, Janet had said she did not want a repetition of her family of origin, which she described as "mother dominated." Her father was not involved with the children. If, after the birth of the child, Daniel continued to live by the old rule of leading parallel lives, that was in conflict with Janet's desire to have her child's father be part of her daughter's life. Janet's symptoms required Daniel to be at home, where he was very involved with his daughter. But he had clearly stated that he wanted to work more. Was this a situation in which, if Janet began to improve, Daniel would neglect the baby? Was that why she had relapsed after her initial improvement?

One other change took place during this period. Janet hired people to help with the housework. The interesting thing was that the people she hired were young, good-looking men, and they did not do any housework. The men came in 12-hour shifts, seven days a week. When they were there, they essentially waited on Janet. If her symptoms were particularly bothersome on a given day, she would stay in bed, and her "house man" would bring her a glass of water, and even keep her company in her room and read poetry to her. While this was occurring, Daniel would be downstairs working away as if he did not care.

I was not sure whether Janet was doing this because she was trying to provoke Daniel to spend more time with her, or if she was arranging a situation in which she and Daniel could continue to lead parallel lives as husband and wife. Would she be satisfied with the arrangement as long as Daniel stayed involved with their daughter? Would Daniel agree to it?

At every session, Janet continued to complain about how Daniel did not treat her as if anything were wrong with her. I began to think that if Daniel were to change how he dealt with her about her symptoms, she might drop the complaints altogether.

I decided to instruct Daniel to treat his wife's complaints as if they were true.

If Janet were literally as ill as she described, what would that mean she should do, and not do? Should she stay in bed all day? How would he treat her? This was a Milton Erickson strategy.

With the most bizarre symptoms, it often undermines the symptoms if the complaints are taken literally. Erickson was a master at this. A famous Erickson example is a case of a hospitalized patient who insisted he was Jesus Christ. Erickson spoke with him one day and said that the understood that the patient was a carpenter. The patient had to agree. Erickson then put the patient to work doing carpentry (Haley, 1983).

Erickson modified the approach for a couple in a case of a husband who constantly complained of severe heart problems. The couple could not go anywhere because the husband might suffer chest pains. They could not have sex because the husband might have a heart attack. There was nothing physically wrong with the husband, but, as with Janet and Daniel, his complaints managed every aspect of the marriage. Erickson advised the wife to treat the problem as if it were literally true. The next time the husband complained of severe chest pains, the wife was to place literature describing local funeral homes and cemeteries on the coffee table. Since the husband was saying his death was imminent, the wife should respond as if this were literally true (Haley, 1976).

In the Erickson approach, the nonsymptomatic spouse is essentially instructed to treat the symptomatic spouse paradoxically. But the approach should be used with extreme caution. Assuming that symptoms exhibited by a spouse are part of an implicit quid pro quo developed by both, for the nonsymptomatic spouse suddenly to ask explicitly for the symptomatic spouse to have the symptom can often result in fireworks.

I spoke with Daniel alone. We discussed the fact that the couple spent so much energy arguing about to what degree, if any, Janet was physically hampered. Daniel agreed that he was very frustrated and that Janet was hypersensitive to the whole topic. If he even had a wrong look on his face, she would launch into a bitter argument about how he had no compassion for her suffering. I explained that I had an idea as to how he might begin to treat her differently that might help her to improve, and maybe eventually even stop her complaining so much about her condition. He was very interested. I asked him what he thought Janet would have to change if she actually were as ill as she described.

He thought about this a moment, "She would have to change a lot."

"What?" I asked.

"If she were as sick as she says she is, she would probably have to stay in bed most of the time. She should not be taking our child out to play. She should definitely not go up and down the stairs. She would have to change a lot."

"How would you treat her differently?" I asked.

"I am not sure," he said.

"Would you insist that she stay in bed if she really were this ill?" I inquired.

"Probably. As it is, she will say that her back is killing her, and then the next minute, she will be going up and down the stairs or out for a walk, as if nothing were wrong."

This is a common reaction from someone who lives with a person with symptoms, when the symptomatic person's actions do not match his or her complaints. Daniel did not really believe that Janet had anything wrong with her. He worked at home, but he ignored her. Ignoring her communicated his disbelief about her symptoms, and this spurred Janet on to complain more. Because Daniel was working at home, the couple spent all day together in this ludicrous pattern of Janet's limping around the house and Daniel's ignoring her.

Daniel was half accepting of the situation and half not. He presumably worked at home because Janet needed him to. But while at home, he treated Janet as if nothing were wrong. I wanted him to go back to work at his office, but he did not follow that suggestion. Now I was switching. If he were going to stay at home, then he should treat Janet as if she needed him there. I suggested that Daniel treat her as if she were really very ill. That would mean his insisting that she stay in bed and not do anything. He would take care of the baby, he would get Janet anything she needed. I was hoping Daniel would cooperate with directives that focused more specifically on Janet's symptoms. More important, I was pushing Daniel to become more directly involved with Janet. I was asking him to change how he was relating to her. I explained that I thought that if Janet had to stay in bed, it might motivate her to improve. Janet was a very intelligent woman. She would soon become very bored if she had to stay in bed all day. Daniel agreed to try it. I cautioned him that he had to be sincere. If Janet thought he was being sarcastic, she would be very angry and this would not help. He said he understood.

Daniel tried the plan. He changed how he was treating Janet. He became more directly involved with her. He insisted she had to stay in bed, the opposite of what he had been doing. Janet rebelled by doing more. The situation quickly became volatile. Less than two weeks later, Janet called me from a hotel. She said that she and Daniel had had a serious quarrel and she had moved out. I asked her what she wanted, and she said that she wanted him out of the house during the day. He was driving her crazy. She wanted him to go back to working in his office. She did not want him to disappear. She wanted him home sometimes, but she did not need him home all day anymore. This was a huge turnaround, and a clear result of Daniel's getting directly involved with Janet.

I asked Daniel to come in and used the fact that Janet had moved into a hotel to push for a change. I suggested that if all he had to do to save his marriage and settle Janet down was to go back to working out of his office, he should do it. I was assuming that Daniel was grappling with deciding what kind of marriage he wanted now that the couple had a child. By my taking a clear position and pushing him in one direction, he might make his own decision about what he wanted to do. With some reluctance, he agreed to give up working at his house. Within a week, Daniel had packed up his papers and had moved his work back to his office and Janet had moved back home. The house was cleaned up and Janet was pleased. This turned out to be the last major turning point in the case. After Daniel moved back to his office, Janet began a period of steady improvement. She continued to complain about her symptoms and was just as convinced as ever that she had a medical problem, but she began to take better care of herself, became more active with the baby, and started to work one day a week. Gradually, she came to the decision to go back to work on a full-time basis. This was a huge change. After she started working full-time, she dismissed her housemen; since she was gone all day, they were not needed.

At that point, Janet and I assessed her need for continued therapy. She had gained weight, and was paying attention to her health. She was long out of any medical danger related to neglecting herself. She was working full-time and Daniel was working out of his office. She had no suicidal feelings. A nanny provided childcare while the couple was at work, and the mother-in-law visited periodically and interacted with the family as a grandmother. When Janet was home, she played with and took care of the baby.

Two changes involving Daniel contributed to these improvements. First, Daniel was more at ease now that the conflict with his mother had been resolved. His entire family had been in an uproar over the situation and because Daniel was tense about it, Janet was tense as well. Second, Daniel changed how he habitually dealt with Janet concerning her symptoms. Although he still did not believe that she had a medical problem, instead of ignoring her, he urged her to do less and to stay off her feet. This provoked her to improve.

Janet continued to be infuriated with Daniel for his not believing she was ill, and she continued to punish him by constantly complaining about her symptoms. She was not, however, doing bizarre things, such as stripping nude and examining herself to see if her spine was disintegrating. Despite her complaints, however, she no longer was seeing a multitude of doctors several times a week. She saw her primary-care physician about twice a month. This was still abnormal for a woman with no medical diagnosis, but it was a vast improvement.

She asked me if I believed I could get any further with changing Daniel. I thought this was a rather interesting question. I said that I did not think he would ever be totally convinced that she had a medical problem in the absence of a clear medical diagnosis. I asked her how she would assess him as a husband and as a father. She said he was a lousy husband but a good father. She decided she was willing to settle for that. I was not sure that Daniel was happy with the arrangement, however. I remembered his comment about having to "endure what life delivers." But he did not have to be happy, he just had to decide whether or not he was going to accept the arrangement Janet wanted. His continued pursuit of her sexually was apparently his last form of protest, and she countered his sexual pursuit by not completely dropping her complaints. The couple had worked out a new quid pro quo that was far less destructive to both.

Janet then asked another interesting question: "Do you think that if a wife were disabled and could not have sex, it would be all right for the husband to find a mistress? Sex with Daniel is painful [she did not specify whether "painful" meant physically or emotionally]. I really do not want to be fighting him off all of the time. I wish he would just get a girlfriend." My hypothesis was confirmed. She wanted him to be a father to their child. She did not want him to be a husband to her. She wanted to keep the set-up whereby they lived parallel lives as husband and wife, but not as mother and father. She wanted Daniel involved with the child, but not with her. The entire struggle had revolved around that. I wondered whether this might be why Daniel was hesitant about working out of his office. Somehow, doing that would be accepting the arrangement Janet wanted. He had to decide if he was willing to be a father, but not a husband. Apparently, but with reluctance, he had decided to agree.

In response to her question, I said, "There is no right way to have a marriage. Every couple has to work out what rules the spouses want regarding relationships outside their marriage. As far as having sex goes, you shouldn't have to be disabled to say No." She agreed. We both decided it was time to terminate therapy.

An Executive's Wife

A 57-year-old woman came for therapy because of a severe eating disorder. Her psychiatrist had referred the woman to me. The client, Susan, came to our first session alone and explained that she had bulimia, and had had it for the past nine years. During that time, she had been through a variety of treatment programs specifically designed to treat bulimia. She had been in long-term inpatient treatment, long-term outpatient psychotherapy, and extensive group therapy for eating disorders. At the time she began therapy with me, she was on a high dosage of Prozac. It was thought the Prozac would reduce her obsessions with food and with bingeing and purging.

First Session: A Consultation

Susan was a very agreeable woman who gave the impression that she would politely go along with any idea or suggestion offered, but underneath this polite veneer was a determination to do things her way. She was extremely thin. In the first session, she explained that her eating disorder had begun when she and her husband moved to Ohio from St. Louis. Her husband, Bob, was a vice-president in a computer company. After living in St. Louis for many years, the family moved when Bob's company transferred its headquarters to Ohio. The couple had three children, two girls and a boy, all of whom were grown and emancipated at the time of the move to Ohio. The two daughters were married. The son was not. Bob's parents were deceased, as were Susan's parents. She had no siblings.

When the family lived in St. Louis, Bob was very involved with his company and Susan was very involved with raising their children. Although Susan was a certified accountant, she had left the workforce to be a full-time mother. She was a cub scout mom who organized her activities around the interests of her children. When she and Bob moved to Ohio, Susan no longer had the childrens' activities to organize her, and her eating disorders began.

I was very interested in Susan's rituals around her symptoms, and her family's, and particularly her husband's, participation in those rituals. To discover this, I had Susan take me through a typical day, highlighting her eating disorders. She said that typically when she got up, she would eat a small, healthy breakfast, and then work out. For lunch, she would have a salad and yogurt. Sometimes she and her husband lunched together. Mornings and afternoons generally were not problem times regarding bingeing and purging. Dinner, however, was another matter. For dinner,

Susan usually cooked an elaborate meal for Bob, who generally arrived home between 7:30 and 8:00 P.M. The couple would sit down together for dinner and Bob would eat while he read the *New York Times*. While Bob was reading the paper, Susan would begin to binge. Bob continued to read. After bingeing, Susan would politely excuse herself from the table, go into the downstairs bathroom, and vomit. She then would come back to the table. Bob would say nothing, and continue to read.

After dinner, the couple would adjourn to the den with a glass of wine and Bob would recount his day at the office. Susan would listen to Bob's daily litany of work events for the nine thousandth time, politely acting interested. At some point during Bob's recital, Susan would excuse herself again, go to the downstairs bathroom, and vomit again. She might purge once or twice after her vomiting episode during dinner depending on how many snacks she and Bob had had, and on how much Bob's day sounded like his last 9,000 days.

Susan was convinced that Bob was unaware of what she was doing. She described Bob as neglectful, and as parading her around as a corporate wife at his various conventions. She dutifully went along with him on business trips, standing by his side while he and his buddies discussed company matters. Bob had accompanied Susan to some of her previous therapy sessions, where he was confronted by the therapists as being insensitive. Apparently, this did not change anything, except perhaps to make Bob reluctant to accompany Susan to therapy again, a problem I would have to overcome.

Susan was bingeing and purging an average of two or three times a day. On a rare day, she would become obsessed with food early in the day and purge up to 15 times. She would not binge, but she would become so concerned about having eaten too much that she would purge over and over. This happened perhaps once a month. It was not clear what triggered it. Susan's health was a real concern. She had colon problems, which she reported as related to her bulimia. Her weight was obviously low. She had numerous physical ailments related to nine years of bulimia.

My immediate problem, however, was how to avoid being the

27th therapist who had failed to help her. Somehow Susan and I were going to have to rise to the occasion if we really were to solve her problem. Somehow this therapy was going to have to be a different experience for her if I were really going to help. Susan would have to commit to that up front.

I told Susan that I did not want her to consider this a first therapy session. I wanted her to consider it a consultation only. I explained that if she and I were to work together, I would have to be her last therapist. We were going to cure her of the problem or die trying. She was going to have to think over what she would have to do to make me her last therapist. If she wanted a second appointment, I would want her to come back prepared to do three things: to give me permission to call her medical doctor, to bring in her husband, and to maintain a chart showing every time she had binged and purged since the first appointment. Susan seemed prepared to agree to all of this immediately, but I cautioned her not to act too hastily. I told her that she should go home and think it over. If she felt the same after sleeping on it a while, she could schedule a second appointment. On the other hand, if she changed her mind and did not want to work with me, that would be all right.

My thinking was as follows: (1) I wanted to motivate Susan to do whatever it would take to solve the problem, and to set the therapy up in a way that her previous therapists had not. (2) I wanted to establish early on that this would be a therapy in which I would give directives. Having her make a chart is a simple directive to give, but bulimia is a secret sin, so her making a chart for me would be revealing those sins. Typically, a client will begin to improve rather than show a bad chart. (3) My initial hypothesis was that the husband would have to change in some way for the therapy to be successful. The problem was how to include him without blaming him.

Susan called a few days later and said that she wanted to come back. She had spoken with her husband, and although he would be out of town for a few weeks, he did agree to come in. A second appointment was set up with the agreement that her husband would come the next time. She made a chart, which she brought in. She was embarrassed. I also learned more about the family situation. Her only son had serious problems. The oldest child, he had been a drug addict since he had left home, which, coincidentally, was around the time Susan and Bob moved to Ohio. He had returned home numerous times. On the last occasion, he had stolen all of the couple's jewelry and pawned it for drug money. Bob became so angry that he threw the son out of the house. The son then disappeared. Susan was unaware of his whereabouts, and had not heard from him in over a year. She thought he probably still lived in St. Louis. He was now in his early 30s. Susan's two daughters were married, and had young children. They both visited occasionally, and Bob and Susan also visited them. One daughter lived in St. Louis and the other on the East Coast.

Susan had a family doctor who was monitoring her physical condition. She gave me permission to speak with him. She also gave me permission to speak frankly to her husband about whatever I learned from the doctor. I called the doctor after this second appointment. I wanted to be able to give the husband a full report, including her medical condition, when he came in. There would be no secrets about Susan's condition. The doctor was very concerned about her. He explained that she should weigh 20 pounds more for her to be healthy and that her potassium level was too low, which could result in dizziness and fainting. I asked the doctor what a dangerous weight for Susan would be. He said he would hospitalize her if she went below 90 pounds; she currently weighed 91. He checked her weight every other week. The doctor agreed that he would send her to the hospital for medical reasons only. I said that I would provide the mental health treatment, and that I would try to keep her from being hospitalized for mental health reasons. The doctor said he was glad someone else was trying to help.

The Husband Attends

Bob did come to the third session. He was nothing like the man Susan described. She had painted him as pushy, neglectful, and controlling. Bob presented himself as a soft-spoken, unassuming person, who felt guilty about Susan's problem. He sat with his head lower than Susan's during the session. I did not want a repetition of his previous experiences with Susan in therapy, and I explained that I had invited him in as the expert about his wife, and that if I were going to help Susan, I would need his help. I defined the wife as the patient, and her bulimia as the problem, not his treatment of her. I explained that the problem was very serious, and that Susan was on the verge of being in jeopardy physically. I reported what Susan's doctor had told me about the state of her health. Bob was surprised. He did not realize the severity of her illness. Susan had been concealing that from him.

I asked him what he knew of the problem. Bob then recounted, almost word for word, the exact nightly routine that Susan had described earlier. Bob knew everything! But he never said anything! They both pretended that Bob was unaware of Susan's problem. I asked Bob how it affected him personally. He said the greatest effect it had on him was that Susan could not have sex without pain. They had sex far less frequently than before. I asked him at what weight he thought Susan looked her best. Bob said, "Susan is beautiful at any weight." He was patronizing Susan, and she knew it.

I had my diagnosis. Bob was not asserting himself in the most dire of circumstances. It was not that he was controlling and pushy. He was too unassuming. He knew that his wife was wasting away before his eyes, and he did nothing! She would get up from the table to vomit, and he would continue to read the paper! He would take her with him to his conventions, and he would be accompanied by a walking skeleton, but he would not even acknowledge it. Instead, he said she was beautiful at any weight. He could not take a stand. I wondered whether this might be part of a quid pro quo. Why did he not assert himself? The easiest way to find out would be to ask him to assert himself and observe what happened.

During the session, with both Susan and Bob present, I asked what Bob could do that would be helpful. Susan said that she was bored. She missed him, and was tired of doing the same thing every evening. I asked her what she had to look forward to. She said, in a dramatic way, that she had nothing to look forward to. She was very depressed about this. One possibility was that she was worried about Bob. Her complaint could be a metaphor about Bob. He might be the one who was bored and had nothing to look forward to. I asked Susan if she had any women friends. She said when she and Bob moved to Ohio, they joined a country club, but that did not work out. Bob then said that the two of them had never "grown roots" in Ohio. They had been here for nine years and neither one had friends! It was now apparent that Susan was being very protective of Bob. In St. Louis, she had had an active social life. She was not a shy person. It was clear she could make many friends if that was what she wanted. My hypothesis was that Bob was ruled by his work and had no friends. I hypothesized that if Susan were to have a social life, she would feel guilty going out and leaving Bob at home with no one to talk to. Bob was suffering, and so Susan had to suffer also. She had sacrificed her social life for him and was protecting him by not saying so. My problem was how to help Bob while staying in the framework of Susan's being labeled the patient. I feared that if I pointed out that Bob had serious problems, Susan would not cooperate.

I utilized the approach of putting him in charge of helping her. Within this framework, I could ask Bob to do things that not only would help Susan, but would also help him. I asked if he would arrange for them to break their routine and go out more often. I explained that this would help Susan with her problem, since she was bingeing and purging at home every evening. It was also agreed that Bob would go grocery shopping with Susan to make sure that she did not purchase the foods on which she typically binged. He agreed.

To get at the questions of why the couple pretended that Susan was not really vomiting every evening and of why Bob was not asserting himself, I had a special task for Bob. At the end of the session, I spoke to Bob alone, and asked him to do one additional thing. The next time Susan binged at the table, I asked that he simply put down his paper and say to her, "Please don't do that. It's bad for your health." He agreed. How he would react to this directive, and what her response would be if he carried it out, would tell me more about why they had this arrangement, and what to do about it.

After a serious effort to get Bob involved in helping his wife, he basically did nothing. He did go to the grocery store with her a few times, and he did take her out a few times. He never said anything to her at dinner when she was bingeing or purging, however. For several days in a row, he said he tried to bring himself to say something, but he just could not do it. It was as if he had had an existential crisis over whether or not to simply say to Susan that she not binge. Obviously, the no-talking rule was part of their quid pro quo, but it was not yet clear why. In time, Bob's work schedule took over, and he was back to traveling and keeping late hours. I was stuck seeing Susan alone, with Bob accompanying her very infrequently.

I began to think that if I were going to help Susan, it was going to have to be with a strategy that did not include Bob's regular attendance. I worked with Susan for several sessions attempting strategies that would not require Bob's full participation. Using this approach, Susan improved and then relapsed. She then came in complaining about Bob, and said she did not think she could change without more of his help. We were back to square one. It was as if to get Bob involved, we first had to try something without him and have that fail.

Hospitalization and Crisis

Soon after this setback, Susan had to go into the hospital to have part of her colon removed. Both she and her doctor explained that her colon problems were indirectly related to her bulimia. Nine years of eating disorders had taken their toll. We scheduled her next appointment for a few weeks after her surgery. When the date arrived, she called to cancel, saying she needed more time to recover. I became concerned. I had not seen her since before her surgery, and I was worried that she was avoiding me. I feared she was losing weight and that no one was monitoring her. I called her and asked if anyone was checking her weight.

She said, "No." I asked her about her purging. She was not talking to anyone about that either. I asked Susan if it was all right for me to make a home visit. She assented.

I immediately went to Susan's house, an expensive home in an elite suburb. A perfect house for the perfect couple. Susan, looking like a walking skeleton, cheerfully answered the door, and invited me in. She had coffee prepared. I asked her what her weight was. She said, "About 80 pounds." I asked if any of the medical people were aware of it. She said they were not. She said she lost the weight while in the hospital recovering from surgery and the surgeon had released her without conferring with the doctor who was monitoring her weight. I insisted that we call her doctor right then, and I did so with Susan cheerfully drinking her coffee. I explained to him that I was at Susan's home, and that she had told me that her weight was down to 80 pounds. He was very alarmed, and insisted that she be taken to an emergency room immediately. I told Susan what the doctor ordered.

I then called Bob, who was at work. I told him about my conversation with the doctor, and explained that it was a medical emergency. He was to come home at once, and take his wife to the hospital. It was a crisis. I was using the opportunity to up the ante on Bob and make another attempt to motivate him. It was possible that the problem with which Susan came in was not severe enough to cause a real change in the husband. Susan had to get worse first before the husband would begin to change. In looking back, I believe that is what Susan was thinking. Bob came home and took her to the hospital, and I told him that I would meet him there in a day or so.

Before my meeting with Bob at the hospital, I called the physician. His plan was to keep Susan in the hospital until her weight had increased to over 90 pounds. He viewed the current relapse as a product of her not being monitored by the surgeon during her hospitalization for colon surgery, not as a failure of the therapy I was offering. I explained that I was going to use the current crisis to push for major changes. We kept our agreements intact.

I arranged to see Bob in Susan's hospital room. The potential that Susan would seriously harm herself was present, and I was determined that it not occur. I went to the meeting thinking I was going to pull out all of the stops. When I arrived, I found Susan, a cheerful skeleton, and Bob having a pleasant conversation, both busily playing the "nothing wrong here" game. I said to Bob, "Let's take a walk." We found an empty room, and I let him have it. In a true crisis, the therapist has to rise to the occasion. That means making statements that match the intensity of the situation.

I told Bob, "We could be at her funeral right now."

He said, "I know."

I said, "If we were at her funeral, you would be regretting that you did not do more when you had the chance. I don't want to see you faced with that situation."

Bob said, "I know."

I said, "This is it. You have to step up and take charge, whatever it takes. Can I count on you?" An emphatic "Yes" came back.

When a therapy approach is not working, changing the unit is often a powerful strategy. I decided to add people to the therapy unit. I told Bob, "This is what we are going to do. You are going to call all of the children and have them fly out for an emergency session. At that meeting, we are going to make a plan, and you are going to stick to whatever agreements are made. You have to decide what is more important, your work or your wife's life." He agreed to call the two daughters, but said he did not know how to contact his son. A therapist should always be skeptical when family members say that someone in the family cannot be found, or that the family is uninvolved with a client. Experienced family therapists know this is usually not the case, and that if pressed under the right circumstances, "uninvolved" family can be brought in. I suggested that one of his daughters might know how to find his son and that he should put the word out to locate him. He agreed and said he had been giving a lot of thought to the situation and realized that his wife's life was in danger, and that his work would have to take a back seat.

Back in Susan's room, I had Bob explain to her how concerned he was about her and what we were going to do. He told her he was very worried and that he was going to become more involved. She did not believe him. He also told her that he wanted to set up a meeting with all of the children when she got out of the hospital. Susan was incensed at this idea. She was violently opposed, saying she did not want the children inconvenienced. I said that it could not be a secret anymore, and that everyone needed to pitch in and help. Bob hung in there and insisted. Susan then became very angry and said that if we had her drug-addicted son come, she would kill herself. This suicide threat confused me. It made me cautious. I told Susan I would think over what to do and took the position that Bob *was* going to get more involved, and that the children would be notified about a possible meeting.

Mobilizing the Family

In the most serious cases, a therapist will often face crucial decisions. The decision here was whether to press for all of the children to come to a meeting despite Susan's threat of suicide, or to back off and only ask the two daughters. Should I allow a chronically bulimic woman to control the therapy? I decided to take the suicide threat seriously, but to search for a compromise. I pushed for a meeting that would have the two daughters attend. The son would be involved by having his whereabouts clarified, and being informed of his mother's condition. Susan agreed to this.

There were three goals for the family meeting: (1) to elicit ideas from the larger family about what might help; (2) to demonstrate the seriousness of the situation by having everyone fly in from out of town; (3) to motivate the husband. The implicit message would be that Bob was not taking care of his wife. Without even making this point explicit, Bob would be shamed in front of his children for even allowing Susan to deteriorate to such a state.

Susan's weight rebounded to above 90 pounds and she was released from the hospital. Bob called the daughters, and they said they were willing to come. The wayward son was located (magically, in about one week) and told about his mother's condition. He had been homeless and basically was in and out of various friends' homes. Apparently he was a serious alcoholic. Interestingly, after he heard about his mother, and that she was permitting us to make such a major effort to help her, he checked himself into a detox program.

A meeting was set up that would include Susan, Bob, and the daughters and their husbands. The night before the meeting, the son called home and spoke to both parents for the first time in at least a year. He told his mother that he loved her and wanted her to get better. The call meant a lot to Susan. He had broken his silence, and she was touched by what he said.

To begin the family therapy meeting, I apprised everyone of the seriousness of the situation, and had Bob explain the medical risks. I asked if anyone had any ideas about what might help. They all said that they had always known that their mother had an eating disorder but had not spoken to her about it so as not to embarrass her or make her uncomfortable. They had played the same game of pretending that nothing was wrong. They all were very concerned, however, and appreciated the opportunity to come together and talk about the problem. I explained that their mother could have died. They all told her they loved her and wanted her to recover. The older daughter was the most outspoken. She said that her mother had been obsessive about food for years, and that she hesitated to ask her to dinner because of her perfectionist attitude toward food. She said, "How can we have you over for a cookout? How could I give you a piece of grilled chicken? You are so meticulous about food, I would be embarrassed to serve something like that."

I had Bob explain to his daughters what he was going to do to help their mother recover. I wanted him to make a commitment to his children. He clearly had his tail between his legs. He described various ideas we had considered, most of which he had never implemented. No one accused him of being neglectful, however. Instead, the daughters offered some good advice about what he might do. The meeting ended with a commitment from the daughters that if their mother ever again began to deteriorate as she had before her recent hospitalization, they would all come out and stay for as long as it took to solve her problem (Schiff & Belson, 1988). Susan objected, saying that she did not want her problems to interfere with their lives and that they might lose their jobs if they did what was being proposed. With no prompting from me, both daughters said they would do anything to avoid having their mother die and that they would come without hesitation. What this meant to me was that Bob was now answerable to his children if he did not follow through. Susan's life was in Bob's hands. That is how the meeting ended.

Next, I had the couple come to my office. I had given a lot of thought to the case since Susan had been hospitalized. One thing that stood out was that Susan's bulimia had begun when the couple moved to Ohio. She did not have eating disorders in St. Louis. What was it about this move? Another thing that stood out was that Susan emphasized being depressed. She said she had nothing to look forward to. They were at a stage in life where Bob's retirement was imminent. What Susan had to look forward to was a few more years of a boring life with Bob working for his present company, followed by his retiring and having nothing to do. As a way to organize the couple, I decided to shift my gears and emphasize Bob's impending retirement. What were the couple's plans? Where would they live? What would they do together? Could I use the upcoming life-cycle transition to get them to make changes?

I started this session with Bob alone. I asked him, "At what weight do you really find your wife the most attractive? Don't give that she is beautiful at any weight crap."

"Well, she's her most attractive at around 115 to 120 pounds," he answered.

"OK, when she comes in, you are going to tell her that," I replied.

I had to be hard on Bob or I would lose the case. This was awkward, because Bob was my senior. He was an older, and in many ways wiser, man than I, but I had to jump all over him about how to deal with his wife. One way I balanced this out was to seek his financial advice. Bob was knowledgeable about mutual funds. I was not, and needed to be. I often asked his advice on this topic, and he enjoyed giving me ideas. Our relationship allowed him to have some dignity in relation to me at times when I had to be hard on him.

I brought Susan into the room and talked to them both about their future. I asked about Bob's retirement, what his plans were. Susan erupted. She said he had no plans, and when his retirement suddenly hit him, he would not know what to do. I said to Bob that this was a problem, especially since Susan was depressed and complained of having nothing to look forward to. She should be able to look forward to plans for the future and be pleased by what they had in mind. I suggested that they get busy planning. They would have to decide where they wanted to live, and what they both would be doing. Would Bob work at all? If so, how much and doing what? They agreed that they would not stay in Ohio, and that Bob would probably continue to work, but much less, and in a job that did not require travel. I suggested that the first task then was to decide where they would live. This would require them to take trips together and to explore new cities. First, however, they would have to decide if they wanted to return to St. Louis. Susan loved the idea of traveling to new cities and planning where they would live next. She said she no longer wanted to live in St. Louis, however. They agreed that they would go on four trips together in the next 12 months. Susan was very excited about this idea.

At the end of the session, I asked Bob to tell Susan at what weight he thought she was her most attractive. He nervously said she looked her best at 115 to 120 pounds. Susan said she knew he was lying before, and appreciated his honesty.

A Breakthrough

After this session, big changes started to take place. Bob became much more active. He came to sessions and he stuck to what he said he would do. The couple planned several trips together over the next several months. First they went on a one-week vacation just to relax. Susan reported that while vacationing, she had no bouts with her eating disorder. She did not binge. She did not purge. She said it did not even occur to her to do so. When she came home, however, she went back to bingeing and purging, although at a very reduced rate. It looked as though she were willing to trade her symptoms for a more meaningful marriage.

Things continued to improve until the couple went on a trip to Arizona. This was their first trip to survey an area to which they thought they might like to move. When they came back, Susan had a major relapse. She had one of those terrible days in which she was obsessed with purging. She said she purged 20 or more times that day. I asked how the trip went. She said it was terrible. She said that she was very excited about the area and thought they could be very happy living there and they began to look around at neighborhoods and condos. She said Bob was not enthusiastic, however. He said all the right things, but he acted as though he was uninterested. Susan became distraught, thinking that he had just been going through the motions with all his latest changes and promises. Of course, she said nothing to him. She just came home and vomited. It was clear that Susan's way of communicating her displeasure with Bob was by bingeing and purging. She would protest by vomiting, not by speaking.

This relapse was followed by a period of Bob's being in and out of town and so unavailable for therapy for several weeks. Susan was making her complaints about Bob explicit to me. She refused to entertain the idea of making her complaints explicit with Bob, however. It was a classic double bind. She wanted Bob to spontaneously want their marriage to change. To demonstrate this to her, she wanted him to take the initiative. If she made her wishes known to Bob, however, Bob would patronize her and seemingly comply. Susan would then believe that Bob would not be complying because he wanted to, but because she was requesting it.

Susan's physical condition was still shaky and she could hardly stand any more days of bingeing and purging 20 times. Since she did not like to tell Bob anything, I suggested she improve in secret. I asked how much weight she could gain before Bob would notice. She said about five pounds. I then suggested she could gain up to five pounds, and cease her bingeing and purging and not tell Bob. She could secretly improve. Every evening that Bob was home, she could get up from the table as always, go into the bathroom, and just flush the toilet. She did not have to actually vomit. Bob would just think that she had. She could express her displeasure about the situation, but not hurt her body. She could pretend to be bulimic. She thought this was ridiculous. I insisted there were no better alternatives. She had already proved her reluctance to improve without Bob's improving. She could not continue to binge and purge without doing terrible harm to her body, and she was unwilling to express her complaints to Bob verbally. The only thing left was to continue to act as though she were sick but she did not have to actually be sick. She did not like this idea and left upset.

At the next appointment, Bob unexpectedly showed up alone. He explained that Susan had insisted he do so. He described the trip to Arizona, maintaining that, despite Susan's impression to the contrary, he was not unenthusiastic about the idea of moving there. He went on to say how frustrated he was at trying to please Susan. He did all that she asked but she still was not satisfied. I asked him if they liked to dance. He said that at one time, they had really enjoyed ballroom dancing.

"Who would lead?" I asked.

Bob said, "I would, of course."

"That is what you have to do now," I replied.

The only way for Bob to escape the "be spontaneous" paradox would be for him to take the lead and initiate something for which Susan had not asked. He was so busy patronizing her that doing this would never occur to him. He was always waiting for her to indicate to him what he was to do. Because he never initiated anything, Susan was left wondering what he really wanted. Did he really want to move to Arizona or was he just going along with her? This question was what was upsetting Susan.

I sent Bob home with the directive to surprise Susan and do something that she would find out of character for him. It could be something that would please her or something that would bother her, it did not matter which, as long as she would find it out of character. We talked about some possible examples, and the session ended. The next week, Bob came back alone. He told me that he had decided to surprise Susan by taking her on a trip to New Orleans for their anniversary. Their date was a month away and they had never done anything like this before. He planned to keep her totally in the dark right up until they had to get on the plane. I thought this was a wonderful idea, and encouraged him.

I did not see either of them again until after their trip. Susan came in alone. She was transformed. She was so surprised by Bob's idea and so pleased. She recounted the whole story. Bob had told her to pack her bags but did not say what was going to happen until they were boarding the plane. He had a great weekend planned that included the theater, dinners at fancy restaurants, and a stay in a luxury hotel. It was totally out of character for Bob. Susan was convinced he really was changing. I asked her about her bulimia. She said she no longer knew why she still binged and purged. It was now like a bad habit that had no reason for being. It was drastically reduced, and for the first time since the problem began she felt as though she would be able to overcome it totally.

One month later, the spouses came in together. Susan was not bingeing or purging at all. Bob had notified his CEO that he wanted a new position in the company at its Arizona location. He did not want a position that would require travel, and he wanted to move within the year. Susan was very pleased. More important, they were doing more together. They were volunteering at a local theater, and were socializing more. Susan said, "It's like we are best friends again. We can talk to each other again." I saw the couple three more times, spacing the appointments at six-week intervals. Susan still was able to report that she had not binged or purged. The couple continued to progress and looked forward to moving. We all agreed there no longer was a need to meet.

A Relapse

Six months passed. I heard nothing. Then a call came from Susan. She requested an individual appointment, saying problems had started again. She came in and said she and Bob had lost their friendship. They were not connected and she was again beginning to binge and purge. She wanted to try to solve the problem before it got worse. I asked about their plans to move and for Bob to scale down his career. She said the plans had changed. They were not moving to Arizona. Bob did take a different position, and they were moving, but to Denver instead. She was very disappointed. She and Bob were no longer volunteering together, no longer socializing. The friendship she felt they had rediscovered had been frittered away. When I asked how this happened, she gave a vague answer. She was again bored and filling her time with obsessions about food. The spouses were back to talking only about Bob's work. Yes they were moving, but Susan was anticipating a continued life of being a "corporate wife."

I prodded for Susan to communicate openly with Bob, something she was not doing. Susan wanted to "retire" from the job of corporate wife. She hated that role, but she would not assert herself and tell this to Bob. It was all they had connecting them to each other. I told her that the difficulty here was that Bob wanted to keep her as a corporate wife, and she did not want to be one, but she was not negotiating. She should negotiate. If he wanted her to accompany him to a conference and to parade her around as his wife, it should cost him. She should insist on something in return. If he wanted to sit around in the evening and talk about work, it should cost him. What would she want in return? How about a trip to New York in return for a "corporate wife" trip? She said that would be wonderful. I asked if that would be an acceptable alternative to vomiting. She said, "Yes." I asked for her permission to let me help her negotiate these issues with Bob.

I had to get Bob in again, but I needed a new framework. I had to change my approach again. I decided to take responsibility for the relapse. I had not stuck with the partners long enough for them to complete their plans and solidify the changes they had made. I apologized to Susan for that. I told her that I would need to see Bob alone, and that I would apologize to him as well.

Before seeing Bob, I gave great thought to what might have happened. Several things were possible. The worst possibility was that after improving their marriage, one or both may have concluded that a void still existed, even with an improved marriage.

One of them may want out of the marriage. Here, Bob would be the obvious candidate. Rather than saying this aloud, however, they just returned to their old pattern. Also, I had failed to inquire into their sexual relationship. Bob mentioned early on that their sexual relationship was an unsatisfactory aspect of their marriage, and I was not sure whether it ever improved, even after they had became closer. It was very possible that Bob simply did not find Susan attractive. A third possibility was that Bob was in a triangle with his wife and his superior at work. He might have had a boss who pulled him back into his work at the time that Bob was attempting to pull out. My plan was to see Bob alone, probe him about these possibilities, and then bring the partners in together.

Bob agreed that they had lost the closeness that they had achieved earlier. But he insisted that he still loved Susan and found her attractive. I asked him if, during the time their marriage had improved, their sex life had improved also.

He said, "Our sex life improved immensely. The intimacy was dramatically better."

I asked him why he thought things had deteriorated recently. Susan was vague on this point; Bob was very clear. Bob said Susan was disappointed because he took a different job than he and Susan had discussed, and they were now moving to Colorado instead of Arizona. When I asked him why he had changed his job plans, he said his CEO had pressured him to. Bob was caught between his boss and his wife. His actions suggested that his loyalties were with his boss.

I now was beginning to understand. Bob had made a unilateral decision nine years earlier when the couple moved from St. Louis to Ohio. Susan countered with multiple forms of silent protest. She silently vomited, and she silently protested with the restrictions she placed on their sex life. The quid pro quo was: "If you are going to let work rule our lives, I am not going to make you happy." Bob was not in a position to assert himself when Susan vomited at dinner because he knew, after he made her move to Ohio, that he deserved what he was getting. Now he was making the same mistake again. I explained that I was worried that he was not negotiating with Susan on these work issues and that he was setting himself up for problems again. He was very open to this and insisted that his marriage was more important to him than his work. I told him he might be thinking that privately, but he was not acting as though he meant it.

Complete Recovery

One week later, Susan and Bob came in together. Susan looked very bright, and Bob had a big smile. They explained they had solved everything on their own. They had a discussion about where they should move and what work Bob should do. Susan asserted herself and insisted that a move to Denver did not make sense since they both wanted to end up in Arizona in a few years anyway. They should just move to Arizona now. After lengthy discussions, Bob agreed with Susan. They went back to their original plan. They were going to move to Arizona, and Bob would take the job that required less travel. Bob seemed genuinely satisfied with this decision. He admitted that his boss had pressed him to rethink his earlier decision, and that his loyalty now needed to be with Susan, not his boss. This represented a very significant change. The couple negotiated aloud instead of developing an implicit quid pro quo, as they had done in the past and Bob asserted himself with his boss. He had to put his loyalty with his wife.

Interestingly, Bob volunteered the information that their son was getting married. Apparently, for the past year, since Susan had been hospitalized, the son had been improving on his own. After entering a detox program, he had been sober for almost a year. He was working as a carpenter and was getting married. This was the first time he had ever proposed to a woman. The son's improvements paralleled those of his mother. Both Susan and Bob were very encouraged by this. I do not know to what degree, if any, Susan's improvement influenced the changes their son had made. I do know that of all of her children, Susan was closest to her son.

Before the couple left, I asked to see Susan alone. I asked her if she was satisfied with what she had negotiated with Bob. She said she was very satisfied and that she was looking forward to moving to Arizona and retiring from her role as a corporate wife. Her bulimia had stopped again. Before she left, she told me how Bob's transfer from St. Louis to Ohio had transpired. The company executives, which included Bob, were told that the firm's headquarters would be moving to Ohio. Bob came home and announced that the family would have to move. Susan pointed out that two or three other executives were not moving, but were leaving the company and would try to find work in St. Louis. Bob replied, "We have to go where they put the food on the table!" They moved to where the food was put on the table, and Susan spent nine years vomiting it right back up.

Follow-up

Over the next nine months, I heard twice from Susan. She sent me a postcard several months after they had moved saying she was doing very well and was very excited about their new location. Most interesting though was her comment about Bob. She said that the most rewarding thing about the move was seeing the smile on Bob's face when he came home. Bob was happy. This was what Susan emphasized.

Finally, I received a Christmas card, on which Susan again said that she and Bob were doing very well. She wrote that she, Bob, and their daughters and their families had all spent Christmas at the home of her son and his new wife in St. Louis. She gave no further explanation, and I needed none.

6

Absent Fathers

The phenomenon of fathers being under- and/or uninvolved with their children and/or families has become a major sociological theme in our culture (Blankenhorn, 1995), as have the detrimental effects of their absence (Biller, 1981a; Hetherington, 1978, 1985; Lamb, 1986, 1989). In contrast, researchers have increasingly recognized that fathers play a key role in their children's development (Biller, 1981b; Lamb, 1981, 1986; Kotelchuck, 1981; Parke & Sawin, 1976; Radin, 1981, 1983). The larger cultural aspect of this phenomenon is beyond the scope of this book; however, we all know of cases in which a child exhibits symptoms that are coincidental with the child's father either being underinvolved with the child, or having a weak voice in dealing with the child's difficulties. I would like to address this issue as it relates to families who seek therapy for their children.

Getting fathers to participate in the therapy of one of their children has long been viewed by family therapists as a problem. Berg and Rosenblum (1978) conducted a national survey of 60 family therapists regarding the father's participation in child therapy and found that fathers were less likely to call to request treatment for a child, were frequently absent from sessions, and were typically responsible for cancellations. These findings were replicated by Heubeck (1986). Budd and O'Brien (1982) report that only 13% of fathers participated in their parent training for children with behavior problems over the 11-year period 1970–1981.

A crucial question would seem to be whether the father's participation makes a difference in the outcome of child therapy. Gurman and Kniskern (1978) conclude: "The father's presence clearly improves the odds of a good outcome in child therapy" (p. 750). Carr (1998) reported that the participation of fathers in therapy for one of their children has been consistently shown to enhance the effectiveness of treatment, and if the fathers do not attend, it is more likely that the family will drop out of treatment or that the therapy will not be successful. In a review of the literature, however, Heubeck (1986) reported inconsistent findings. He cites several studies showing that the father's participation in child treatment and parent guidance has a positive effect on outcome, but contrasts this with claims from therapies such as the MRI Strategic approach that good outcome has been obtained by working only with the "primary complainant," usually the mother. From his review of the literature, Heubeck concluded that in cases of mild child disturbances, working with only the mother can be effective, but when working with more severely disturbed youths, the father's participation in the treatment is more crucial. Heubeck also concluded that when including fathers in treatment, good outcomes are obtained when the fathers are asked to carry out specific tasks, such as taking more responsibility for disciplining the problem child, spending more quality time with the problem child, and supporting the mother's parenting of the child.

Confirming Heubeck's findings is one of the more famous family therapy studies conducted by Stanton and Todd (1982). Stanton and Todd provided 10 outpatient family therapy sessions to 43 adult chronic heroin addicts and compared the outcome of this group with a second group of 43 adult addicts who received inpatient treatment followed by intensive outpatient treatment. In the family therapy group, a major emphasis was on getting the fathers of the addicts to participate in the therapy. Despite the fact that many of the addicts described themselves as uninvolved with their fathers, 71% of these fathers came to the first session. Stanton and Todd followed both groups of addicts at six-month intervals for two years after treatment was terminated. The therapy outcome of the addicts from the family therapy group showed a statistically significant superiority over that of the addicts from the second treatment group.

A case in which I supervised from behind a one-way-mirror offers a dramatic example of how the mere presence of a father in a family interview made a major difference in the behavior of a child during the therapy session, and in how the case was viewed by the professionals involved. A young mother brought her only child, a 4-year-old son, to their first therapy interview. The problem was that the son was very hyperactive. During the interview, as she recounted all of the parenting techniques she had learned from different professionals and had attempted in vain with her son, the boy crawled all over the floor and was constantly active. No matter what the mother tried during the session, he would not respond to her instructions to sit still. As several of us observed the session from behind a mirror, one participant, a pediatrician, strongly urged that the son be referred to a doctor and be put on Ritalin. I was responsible for the case, and was reluctant to make such a referral after only one interview, especially considering that the boy's father was not present. The session ended with the advice to the mother to invite the child's father to the next appointment, much to the consternation of the observing doctor.

The family returned with the father. The doctor, who was again observing from behind the mirror, was stunned by what he observed in this second session. Both parents sat and discussed their son, while the boy played quietly, and patiently, at their feet. The boy appeared to have no hyperactivity with his father present in the room. The son's behavior had changed dramatically just by including the father in the interview. The father explained what his wife was reluctant to talk about. She had epileptic seizures, and there were times in which she had gone into convulsions when she and the son were at home alone together. Because of this, the boy was very insecure when alone with his mother. Had we followed the advice of the doctor, the boy would have been diagnosed as having ADD, put on medication, and a serious child safety issue that the mother was reluctant to talk about would have been overlooked. Instead, we urged the couple to have a family member stay at home with the mother when the father was absent, to ensure the child's and mother's safety until the seizures could be brought under control. The couple followed this advice, and the boy settled down.

When a child is brought to therapy exhibiting some kind of emotional or behavioral symptom, and the child's father is uninvolved with the child, or is not asserting himself regarding the child's difficulties, in the approach offered here, it is assumed that the father's lack of participation is a product of a quid pro quo between the parents. The parents as a couple develop a rule that defines the father's level of participation. When this type of rule develops, and a child is exhibiting symptoms, an inappropriate relationship may exist between the child and one of the parents. The problem child ends up in a coalition with one parent against the other.

A couple can work out an arrangement in which a particular child is the mother's to deal with. The father is to stay out of it. This is not necessarily a problem, but sometimes it coincides with a distant relationship between the spouses, as well as a relationship between the mother and child as one in which the child becomes the mother's confidant. If the child develops problems, the mother is then in a weakened position to deal with the child with authority. She may want the father's help with the child's problem, but this then would be breaking the rule that the father is to stay out, a rule that both the mother and father created together. In this arrangement, it is typically the mother who brings the child to therapy and the therapist must decide whether and how to include the father. If the therapist does not press for the father's involvement in the therapy, the father may stay in the background, the arrangement the couple has developed may remain unchanged, and the chances for the therapy to be successful may be diminished.

On the other hand, sometimes a problem child is in a special relationship with the father. The father and mother are distant from each other, and one of the children, say, a daughter, becomes very close to the father. If the daughter develops problems, the father may be reluctant to assert his authority with her because of their special relationship. This type of arrangement can result in a hostile relationship between the mother and daughter, particularly when the daughter reaches adolescence. The mother and daughter can end up having chronic, very hostile and destructive arguments, and these arguments are the most noticeable aspect of the arrangement. If professionals become involved, the hostility between the mother and daughter can easily become the focus of the intervention since this aspect of the family is the most obvious. What can be missed is the father, who is in the background, not asserting himself when the mother and daughter get into fights. The intensity and hostility between mother and daughter makes the father's passive contribution less noticeable.

What follows are two case examples of what I believe are common adolescent problems brought to the attention of professionals. The first case is that of a violent teenage son whose father is unavailable to the family owing to his working very long hours. The second case is that of an out-of-control teenage daughter and a father who does nothing when she becomes out of control. In both cases, the characteristic of the father's absence is assumed to be a result of a quid pro quo, and the interventions offer ways to resolve the child's difficulties by, in part, changing this quid pro quo, and thus changing the father's role with regard to the child.

Case 1: A Workingman's Son

> Note: Eugene Bell, M.A. was the therapist in the following case. Although I consulted with Mr. Bell throughout the case, providing suggestions, and helping him plan interviews, it was his skillful handling of the case that resulted in the outcome. The case is presented with his permission.

Fifteen-year-old Darren lived with his father, his mother, and his 21-year-old sister in a small rural town in western Ohio. Darren's father worked 10 hours a day, seven days a week, as a local delivery truck driver. His mother was a full-time homemaker. One day, proclaiming that he "could not take it anymore," Darren arranged for his girlfriend to meet him with her father's car at a secret location so that they could run away. It was not clear what had upset Darren to the point that he "could not take it anymore."

Before meeting with his girlfriend, Darren first paid a visit to his 79-year-old paternal grandmother, demanding that she give him all of her money. When she refused, Darren tied her to a chair and stole all of the money he could find in the house. He then went to meet his girlfriend, but the girl's father somehow had discovered that the two were up to something and called Darren's father. Darren's father called the police, and before the two teens could get away, they were apprehended and it was learned that Darren had tied up his grandmother and taken her money.

Charges were pressed, and Darren was put on probation and ordered to wear an electronic monitor on his ankle so that his whereabouts would be known at all times. He was given a battery of psychological tests and proclaimed sociopathic with a very poor prognosis. The court then referred him for in-home therapy with Gene Bell. Gene was reluctant to take the case in view of the severity of Darren's problems and the pessimism of the court's psychological evaluation. The author, who was consulting with Gene, persuaded him to take it, however, on the basis that there were no better treatment alternatives available in the area. Gene agreed. In listening to Gene describe the presenting problem, the obvious question seemed to be: Where was the boy's father in all of this? It was the paternal grandmother the boy assaulted. What did his father do about this? It seemed as though the man were nonexistent. If this were true, a major change would be to get him more involved with his son. Doing this might make a big difference, especially since the problem involved violence.

Gene began by meeting with the family and Darren's probation officer in the family's home. The probation officer spelled out the legal situation, including what Darren needed to do to have the electronic monitor removed and what would happen to him if he committed any crimes while on probation. During the meeting, Darren's mother, Alice, spoke almost the entire time. William, Darren's father, said very little. He spoke only if Gene asked him a direct question, and then not without first looking over at his wife.

When the discussion turned directly to what Darren had done, his mother minimized the seriousness of his crimes. With regard to Darren's tying up his grandmother, Alice pointed out that it could have been worse, Darren could have gagged her. Alice went on to say that Darren's grandmother "was hard to get along with," implying that she deserved her fate. Gene then learned that the family had little contact with Darren's grandmother because Alice did not like her and forbade her husband to interact with his mother. It was also learned in this first session that the parents led completely separate lives. Darren's father worked all of the time, and when he got home, he went to bed soon after supper, while Alice stayed up late at her computer. Alice was clearly minimizing Darren's behavior, and it was unclear as to how his father regarded it. This was remarkable considering that it was William's mother whom Darren had victimized.

After this first family meeting, Gene decided to meet privately with the boy to try to understand why he wanted to run away. When one on one, Darren opened up quite readily. He explained that he was running away from his mother. He said that she was the boss in the house and was very rigid about allowing him to have any freedom. Darren also said that his mother wanted him to be her best friend. She talked to him about her personal affairs, and this made Darren uncomfortable. Alice was so dependent on Darren that she discouraged him from having a normal social life for a boy his age. For example, when he turned 13, he wanted to play basketball with his friends at a nearby basketball court. Alice did not want him to be away from home, so she had Darren's father put up a basketball hoop in their yard so Darren could stay at home and have his friends over to play.

Apparently, Darren's sister was equally upset with Alice and felt trapped at home, like Darren. At one point, Alice and her daughter were discussing the father of the daughter's infant and his lack of support. Alice told her daughter that she did not need the baby's father, that she had her "mommy." Alice was enmeshed with Darren, and it was driving him crazy. When Gene asked Darren about his father, Darren responded simply and cryptically, "He works." This was the classic problem-child, enmeshed-mother, peripheral-father family structure.

Gene next met with Alice individually. Alice was reluctant to talk to Gene at first, but Gene was determined to get closely connected to her. He knew that for him to be successful in the case, he was going to have to put some distance between Darren and his mother, and that this would be an extremely difficult thing to ask of Alice. To change an organization, one goes to and through power (Haley, 1994). Alice was the powerful person in the family. To have a chance at helping, Gene was going to have to win Alice over. It took several individual meetings with Alice, but gradually she did begin to open up. She admitted to Gene that her children were her whole life.

Early in the case, a court date was set to review whether Darren could have his electronic monitor removed. Both parents and Gene went to court. When the judge asked the parents what they thought, Alice said she thought the monitor should stay on. In her view, Darren did not need to go anywhere anyway. The judge then asked Gene what he thought, and Gene recommended that the monitor come off. Alice was very nervous about this recommendation, but Gene used the rapport he had established with Alice to reassure her. The judge followed Gene's recommendation. This was a major turning point in the case. First, with the ankle monitor restraining him, it was unclear as to whether Darren was truly improving. Improvement would mean Darren's restraining himself, not the court restraining him. Equally important was the fact that the judge followed Gene's recommendation. This demonstrated to the family that Gene had influence with the court and empowered him in their eyes.

It is crucial for therapists to have this type of influence in cases of compulsory therapy. In this case, the parents did not seek the help of a therapist for their son, and Darren himself was not requesting therapy. From the family's viewpoint, the court was intruding into their lives. In a situation such as this, a therapist can offer to advocate with the court on behalf of the client. This then becomes a contract with the family. The therapist can take the position that the client and family take certain steps in order for the therapist to be in a position to advocate on their behalf. The contract becomes: "You follow my recommendations, and I will advocate for you." This contract fails if, when the therapist advocates, the judge does not follow his or her recommendations. Gene did not have this problem.

After court, Gene knew he had to get William involved in both the therapy and his son's life. One way to help Darren and his mother separate would be for Darren to be more involved with his father. This strategy required the mother's cooperation to be successful. The first step to having William become more involved, therefore, was to obtain Alice's permission for William to be more active with Darren. Gene again met with Alice privately. He approached the topic by pointing out that she did everything in the family. She did all of the parenting. If there were problems, she had to be the one to step in. She began to cry, saying that she was very overwhelmed. "Don't you want any help with anything?" Gene inquired. Alice said that she did want help. Gene offered, "Let me get you some help from your husband. Let me put him to work." Alice gave her approval.

Gene then began meeting with both parents. The issues at hand involved how much freedom Darren should have now that his ankle bracelet was off, and what he should do to make amends to his grandmother. It was decided that William would take Darren to his grandmother's house and insist that Darren apologize to her. This idea was obvious but for this family it was outrageous. First of all, it involved breaking the rule that William was not allowed to associate with his mother. More important, it also would mean that William actually was going to take a hand in directly dealing with his son. Despite the fact that they would be breaking their pattern, both Alice and William agreed to the idea.

The more difficult task was persuading Alice to allow Darren to have more freedom. Gene was able to get her to agree on the basis that Darren resented her imprisoning him. Alice did not want her son to hate her. Gene had to press Alice to concede that Darren was doing better and that to avoid causing him to resent her, Darren had to be permitted to have more freedom.

Gene then prodded both parents to communicate more with each other about Darren. He set up a special ritual for them.

They were to go into their bedroom together at a set time each night, close the door, and discuss how Darren did that day. Gene explained that it was important for them to be mysterious to Darren. If they were mysterious, they would be more unpredictable and Darren would be less likely to take the chance of being defiant.

All of these interventions were followed. William took Darren to his grandmother's house and made him apologize. The parents did go into their bedroom and have private talks. Darren was dumbfounded. He could not believe that his parents actually would talk about him behind closed doors. Instead of his mother's having secrets with him about his father, his father and mother were now having secrets with each other about him. Darren was also impressed that his dad had made him apologize. There was a human being inside his father's body after all! As a reward for apologizing, William then agreed to take a computer class with Darren. William now not only was involved with Darren as a disciplinarian, but was also associating with him in positive ways.

Predictably, there came a relapse. Gene was succeeding at getting some distance between Alice and Darren and at getting William more directly involved with Darren. Darren and Alice responded to this by once again attempting to have a secret between them. One day, Alice upset Darren and Darren threatened to kill his mother. Alice told him that he did not mean it, and Darren insisted that he did. In a private meeting with Gene, Alice mentioned Darren's threat almost in passing. Gene was very alarmed. If Darren was capable of tying up his 80-year-old grandmother, he was most certainly capable of being violent with his mother. Gene told Alice that they would have to tell William about the threat and the three of them would have to decide how to handle it. Alice insisted that the threat be kept a secret from William. Gene was equally insistent. He told Alice that he wanted to have a family meeting at his office, where the secret would have to be brought out. Gene decided to punctuate the therapy by not allowing this boundary around Alice and Darren. He had them come to his office (the therapy was being conducted in their home) to emphasize his point.

At the appointed time, Darren and both parents arrived at Gene's office. Gene started with Alice and William and left Darren in the waiting room. Alice then announced to Gene that she had already told William of Darren's threat to kill her. William confirmed this and did not seem overly concerned. Gene spent the next 15 minutes needling William and turning Darren's threat into an act of disrespect toward William. "Darren obviously thinks you are not man enough to defend his mother," Gene pointed out. When William became agitated, Gene called Darren in. When the boy sat down, William told him he knew what Darren had said to his mother, and that he (William) had better never find out that Darren ever said anything like that again. Again, Darren was dumbfounded. First of all, his father was actually angry, and was actually defending his mother! Second, his mother had obviously told on him.

This meeting was followed by a period of great improvement. Darren's grades at school began to get better, his parents were rewarding him with more freedoms, which he was not mishandling, and he was not as unhappy with his mother as he once had been. At some point during this period, Gene had a meeting with William alone at which the issue of William's not seeing his mother was raised. Gene dealt with the matter in an indirect manner. He did not give William advice, but just noted in passing, "You mean you let your wife dictate to you that you cannot associate with your mother!" Soon after this meeting, Darren mentioned to Gene that, to his astonishment, his mother suddenly was allowing his father to visit his grandmother.

Although Darren was improving, he had developed a reputation at school of being violent. This reputation caught up with him when one of the kids started a rumor that Darren had told his older sister that he was going to beat her up. Gene caught wind of this rumor and called a family meeting to deal with it. At the meeting, Darren's sister said that the rumor was not true, that Darren had not threatened her. William was not satisfied with this, however. With no prompting from Gene, William spontaneously looked Darren right in the eyes and very strongly told him that there would be no more threats. Darren had never seen his father so firm. On top of this, Alice was silent. She did not try to dominate the meeting, nor did she criticize William for taking a stand with Darren. The significance of this meeting can be seen when comparing it with the first meeting Gene had with the family. At that meeting, Alice did all of the talking and William was invisible. Now, William was making his presence felt and Alice was accepting it.

Darren's improvement continued, and major changes were occurring in the family. Darren's sister and her infant moved out of the house and into their own apartment. The sister's emancipation was a clear sign that things were getting better. After nine months, Gene felt he could stop seeing the family. Then the final relapse came. Darren's probation officer called Gene and reported that Darren had been caught sneaking out of his house at 1:00 A.M. It was a probation violation and Darren would have to go to court. The judge again asked for Gene's recommendations and Gene advised that the court not handle it like a criminal offense, but let the parents take care of it within the family. Once a youth has been placed on probation, it is common for juvenile courts to use court-mandated punishments for routine adolescent misbehavior, such as sneaking out of the house. This depowers the parents in a situation in which the parents' power is being emphasized. Gene blocked this, and it was helpful that the judge trusted Gene's judgment.

Gene then met with the parents to help them to decide how they wanted to punish Darren. Next, Gene met with Darren privately and Darren had something very important to report. He told Gene privately that his mother had told him that his father was going to leave the family. As Haley (1997) has pointed out, one parent's threatening to leave is a classic reaction to the improvement of a triangulated young person. Darren had improved, and his sister had been emancipated. Now the mother was telling Darren that his father was threatening to leave.

Gene met with the parents together and asked them about this. Apparently, they had a fight and William did threaten to leave. William denied to Gene that he was serious about leaving, but he did express his dissatisfaction with living for years so emotionally distant from Alice. The partners had had no life as a couple for a very long time. Gene was concerned that William might be minimizing the degree of his upset. Gene then took the position that Darren's improvement was too tenuous for him to tolerate having any knowledge of his parent's problems. Gene made Alice promise not to mention anything private about her marriage to Darren at the risk that it might provoke her son to do something that could get him into trouble. If Alice wanted someone to talk to about personal problems, she could call Gene. Gene then asked both parents to start spending more time together. He told them that he did not care whether or not they actually wanted to, but they should give Darren the impression that they were all right. For Darren's sake, they should try to have fun together again. If they found that they could not enjoy each other, to help Darren, they should at least fake it. They agreed.

Alice and William did begin to spend more time together. Darren was again shocked, and responded by staying out of trouble. It is not clear that they actually did improve their relationship. But whether they did or not, Darren was kept out of it. Gene continued to see the family intermittently until Darren's probation was over. When Gene terminated with the family, Darren was entering his senior year in high school and the couple was still together.

Discussion

A parent's colluding with a child to keep important secrets from a spouse, especially about the child's misconduct, puts the parent and child in a coalition against the other parent. A parent's confiding in a child about personal and intimate matters regarding the parents' marriage results in the same outcome. Making a child a confidant and special friend places that child in a non-child role in relation to the parent. Once a child is in this role, the parent damages his or her credibility and authority as a parent to that child.

This type of inappropriate relationship typically coincides with a marriage in which one parent is absent. The couple as a unit creates this situation. It becomes a rule, a quid pro quo, that one parent is out, and is replaced by one of the children. With Darren's parents, William had withdrawn and Alice became overly involved with Darren. From William's point of view, the quid pro quo was, "If you want to be totally in charge of the children, rendering my participation pointless, I am just going to go off and work all of the time." From Alice's point of view, it was, "If you are going to just withdraw and be gone all of the time, I am going to make Darren my confidant."

What does not take place in this situation is negotiation. For example, if William felt excluded, instead of resigning himself to this fate, he could have asserted himself with Alice and insisted that he have some input with the parenting. Instead of disappearing, he could have made his presence felt. He did not have to withdraw. By withdrawing, however, he gave Alice all of the power, and Alice did not necessarily want all of the power. She had a teenage son who was violent, and she was having to deal with him with no help from the boy's father. It seems obvious that the presence of a man can help with teenage boys who are struggling to handle the feelings that go with becoming a man. But this means that the father must make his presence felt in helpful ways, and the mother must give him the room to do so.

To break the arrangement Alice and William had created, the objective was for William to become more directly involved with his son and for the parents to cooperate with each other as parents and to work together as a team. In order for such an objective to be attained, two steps need to be taken. First, it must be recognized that the mother in such an arrangement has the power. As the one with the power, if the father is to be more involved, her approval must be obtained. Gene very skillfully accomplished this by first establishing a trusting and empathic connection with Alice, and then appealing to her common sense regarding the needs of her son. Once the mother has given her permission for the father to get more involved, the therapist must get the father more active. Gene accomplished this by using crisis points in the therapy to provoke William and arouse his motivation to be more involved.

Once the father is more involved with the son and the spouses are working together as a team, the boy is moved out of the "special" relationship position with his mother. This can create, as it did in this case, a crisis between the spouses. Typically, that crisis comes in the form of one of the parents threatening to leave. The goal in this situation is not to resolve all of the couple's marital problems, but to keep the child from being caught in the middle of them. Often, if the parents can be focused on each other for a period of time, the child and couple have a chance to adjust to the child's being out of the middle of it, and the family can work out how to have a marriage without the child's intimate involvement. It is our hope that if William and Alice did not improve their relationship, they at least figured out how to keep Darren out of it.

Case 2: A Powerful Daughter

Wendy was 15 and lived with her father, Glenn; her mother, Kathy; and her maternal grandmother. At my request, she came for her first appointment with both of her parents. Less than five minutes into the session, the family revealed the problem. Kathy started the conversation and before she could finish a sentence, Wendy would correct her. Kathy then would retort. Wendy would reply in a hostile tone, and Kathy would come right back with a venomous response. Wendy would snarl with equal intensity, and so on. While the mother and daughter were busy strangling each other, Glenn sat silently.

Wendy was a pretty girl, and Kathy had seen better days. It was apparent that Wendy was the apple of her father's eye. His interest in his wife, however, was not so apparent. I had the distinct impression that Glenn and Wendy were an "item" and Glenn and Kathy were not. It seemed that serious problems with Wendy had begun about a year earlier when she began abusing marijuana and defying her mother. The home became a war zone with Wendy and Kathy as the combatants. As the hostility increased, so did Wendy's defiant behavior. She began to stay out late and to skip school. She found a boyfriend who infuriated Kathy. The whole thing came to a climax during the summer before Wendy's first year in high school. Wendy and her boyfriend broke up, and Wendy stole her father's credit card, took the family car, and was two states away before the authorities caught up with her.

The police brought Wendy home. Her parents had her hospitalized, and filed charges against her in juvenile court. The hospital staff could not make sense of her behavior other than to assume that her father must be abusing her sexually. Although Wendy denied this and gave no overt signs that it was true, the hospital staff proposed this theory to the family, humiliating Glenn and angering Kathy.

Wendy's stay in the hospital overlapped the beginning of the school year, and so when she was finally discharged, she had to start her first year in high school in the middle of the term, with all of her schoolmates knowing she had been in the hospital. Not discovering sexual abuse, the hospital released Wendy with such a negative evaluation that the school system decided to place her in a class for students with severe behavior problems. After her release from the hospital, her mother called me requesting that I work with Wendy on an outpatient basis.

It took much of the first session to arrive at the facts amidst the venom spitting going on between Wendy and Kathy. The two were equally hostile toward each other, with Kathy responding to her daughter more like a competitor in a gladiatorial contest than like a mother. When a therapist is confronted with a parent, particularly a mother, who is responding to a child in this manner, it is difficult to avoid confronting the parent. One's instincts are to protect the child. Certainly, even if one is able tactfully to distract a parent from this type of exchange, it is all too easy to become absorbed in the battle being waged in front of one's eyes. But the more absorbed a therapist becomes in the intense struggle between the mother and daughter, the more the therapist is missing the key figure, the father, who is silently watching the fight. The intense hostility between the mother and daughter makes the father unnoticeable.

At one of their early sessions, Wendy and Kathy arrived and were already fighting in the waiting room and on the way to my office. I asked Glenn what the fight was about. Had I never asked

Glenn direct questions, he might have sat through the entire therapy without speaking more than one sentence. Glenn described an incident that was a portrait of the family's life. When they were walking to their van to come to my office, Wendy rushed ahead and got into the front seat in order to sit next to her father, who always drove. When her parents caught up with her, Kathy told her to move to the back seat. Wendy refused. Kathy explained, for what must have been the hundredth time, that she could not sit in the back because she got car-sick. Wendy still refused to get in the back seat, and they ended up driving to my office with Kathy in the back seat, nauseated. Glenn, of course, said nothing during the entire episode. After he told me this story, I asked Glenn why he did not tell Wendy to shut up and to sit in the back! He looked at me as though it were some sort of trick question, and then said that if he had done so he would have had World War III on his hands. Glenn was not overtly taking any position in the battle between Wendy and Kathy. But by saying nothing he was essentially siding with Wendy. His passivity was communicating tolerance for the way in which Wendy treated her mother.

His silence put him in a coalition with Wendy, and this made Wendy too powerful. She was so powerful that even if her mother suffered car-sickness, Wendy got her way. Kathy's developing symptoms was not enough to neutralize Wendy's power. The interesting thing was that Kathy never complained that Glenn did not support her. She was very protective of him. The partners were quick to point out that in 16 years of marriage, they had never had a serious quarrel. When they told me this, I thought to myself that this was one of those couples that Milton Erickson undoubtedly would have arranged to have a huge fight. Sixteen years, and they had never had a fight! They must have been ready to kill each other. Obviously, all of the hostility was being diverted to the mother and daughter.

Inquiry into the larger family picture revealed that Wendy was even more powerful than it first had seemed. Glenn and Kathy lived in the country, next door to Glenn's parents. I asked what the parents had to say about the situation, and was informed that they were not communicating with the family because they were so perturbed by the way Wendy was behaving. I also found out that Kathy's mother, who had been living with them for just over a year, was elderly and in ill health, and might have to go to one of Kathy's sisters because the tension in the home was becoming too much for her. Wendy's conduct was regulating the emotional, and perhaps geographical proximity of both of her parents and all of the in-laws! Kathy and Glenn, of course, did not admit to having any difficulties with their respective in-laws. When asked, Glenn said he had no problem with Kathy's mother living with them. But even if he was uncomfortable with the arrangement, he did not have to protest. Wendy did it for him, referring to her grandmother as a sick old bitch. And even though Kathy said she would rather live in town than in the country, she was very adamant that she had no problem with living next door to her in-laws. Any tension there might have been between Kathy and her in-laws was taken care of by Wendy, who essentially chased them away.

Wendy was running the whole show. There was no doubt as to who was supposed to sit in the front seat. Wendy sat up front with her father, who did not insist that she move. Glenn and Wendy were in a coalition, and the coalition was implicit. This coalition gave Wendy power, and power always corrupts, especially when a teenager has it. Wendy was not having to face two parents who were jointly setting limits and outlining their expectations. Only one parent, her mother, did that, and because Glenn minimized Wendy's problems by never saying anything, Kathy had to exaggerate her complaints to make up for his minimizing. Not only were the spouses not functioning as a team, but they were exacerbating the situation by trying to prove a point to each other in the way they each dealt with Wendy. Further complicating the problem was their insistence that they were the perfect couple. They never argued and they never disagreed.

To settle Wendy down and resolve the hostility between her and her mother, Glenn would have to come over to Kathy's side. Glenn's coalition with his daughter would have to be broken and the parents would have to act jointly. The problem was their insisting that they had a perfect marriage. They were denying that Glenn was in a coalition with Wendy. I decided to intervene by putting Glenn in charge of Wendy. Putting him in charge would force his hand. If he were in charge, what he approved of and what he disapproved of would be made clear by the way in which he would have to deal with his daughter.

Although putting the father in charge as an intervention has come under attack by some therapists as promoting a patriarchal system, it is an intervention I use frequently to get fathers more involved, and to break up unhealthy coalitions between problem children and either their mother or their father. Despite some therapist's criticism of the technique, I have never had a mother complain about it, especially in cases where the problem was a father/problem-daughter coalition. When I propose it to families, the mothers know that their husbands are not doing enough with the children. The mothers know when their husbands are secretly siding with the children. Typically, when I ask that the father take charge of a problem child, the mother thanks me.

In Kathy's case, she was very pleased that I was asking Glenn to take charge. She actually said that it was about time a counselor realized what was needed. She did not take it as a sociopolitical statement at all. The idea was that if Glenn took charge of dealing with Wendy, he would have to struggle with her, and eventually would become frustrated and distance himself from her. The goal of putting him in charge was to break up his coalition with Wendy and to get him to support Kathy.

I spoke to the couple, without Wendy present, about Glenn's taking charge. Kathy was pleased with my proposal, but when it was presented to Glenn, he was reluctant and nervous about it. After getting an agreement from Kathy that it should be tried, the rest of this session was spent discussing with Glenn what his priorities for Wendy would be. Wendy was then brought into the room, and it was explained to her that for the next few weeks, Glenn would be in charge. Glenn then told her what he wanted her to focus on: respecting her mother, not smoking marijuana, and coming home on time. If she violated any of these rules, she would have to answer to him. I pointed out that this was being done to give her mother a break and to help her and her mother be able to enjoy each other more. Wendy's reaction was interesting. She sneered at her father and told him, "When we get home, you are going to get it!"

The next week, Wendy's behavior had not improved. Kathy said that Glenn was not doing his job. Wendy had come home late and was showing signs of using marijuana, and Glenn had done nothing about it. Glenn agreed that Wendy was not obeying him, but was mystified about what to do. From my standpoint, the positive development was that Kathy was now openly upset with Glenn. The spouses were not pretending to agree. I prompted them to come to an agreement as to what Glenn should do about Wendy's violating his rules. As might be expected, Kathy dominated the discussion, and I had to work to get Glenn to share his thoughts. They reached some agreements but I was concerned that Glenn was still just patronizing Kathy.

My suspicions were confirmed at my next appointment with the family. The results of pushing Glenn to take charge were unexpected and astonishing. Kathy announced that she was moving out of the house and in with her sister, and was taking her mother with her. She explained that while at home, she could not resist the temptation to take over parenting Wendy. Her inability to stay out of the fray with Wendy led to another mother/daughter fight. Infuriated with Kathy, Wendy spray-painted the word "fuck" on her bedroom wall. Privately, I wondered whether this was an act of protest by Wendy or a command given to her parents. After the spray painting, Kathy decided she was leaving to stay out of the way of Glenn's setting limits on Wendy. Glenn had not implemented the punishments they had agreed on in the last session. Now he would have to deal with the painting episode. Kathy felt her presence in the home impeded him from taking charge. She presented this as her way of putting maximum pressure on Glenn to do something. Kathy was not calling it a separation, just a temporary departure to help Glenn. She was taking her mother with her because she did not think it was fair to Glenn for him to have to care for the grandmother in Kathy's absence. Needless to say, Kathy's leaving was not the outcome I was after, but Kathy was determined. I was not able to dissuade her.

Kathy and her mother did move in with Kathy's sister. I saw

this as a serious problem. First, the spouses had separated and were continuing to conceal the real reasons for distancing themselves from each other. Obviously, there was more going on than disagreements about parenting. The wife in a model marriage does not move out just because her husband failed to ground their daughter. Second, Wendy was being used as their reason for separating. This made Wendy even more powerful. The parents were classifying the situation as one in which Wendy basically ran her mother out of the house. This meant Wendy had won. I did not think this arrangement would make it easier for Glenn to set limits on Wendy. As I saw it, the basic problem was that the partners were too distant from each other emotionally, and Wendy was being used as the excuse for that distance. It was not just about parenting; it was also about the marriage. My problem was how to persuade Kathy either to move back home, or to spell out the real reasons for her departure.

First, I called a meeting with Glenn alone. I apologized to him. I explained that the way I understood it, my asking him to take charge of Wendy had raised Kathy's expectations of him. She actually expected him to do something. When he did not, Kathy became agitated and went to her sister's house. I was sorry for that. But, even so, if he wanted Kathy to return, he had better start getting after Wendy.

Then I called a meeting with Kathy alone. I told her that her moving out was something I thought a lot of mothers in her situation fantasized about doing. A lot of parents feel defeated at times and just want to get away and have their freedom. I offered this explanation as a way to help her save face. I went on to outline my concerns about leaving Wendy at home alone with Glenn, as Wendy was viewing it as a victory over Kathy. It was making Wendy too powerful and disempowered Kathy. She agreed with all of this, but did not want to move back home under the present circumstances. I suggested that while she was staying at her sister's house, she and Glenn could have secret dates. Glenn could leave a note for Wendy saying something like, "I went to be with your mother," leaving it vague as to what "being with" meant. Glenn and Kathy could have secret rendezvous. Having the couple date secretly would put a boundary around them. The secret would then be between Glenn and his wife, not Glenn and his daughter. Kathy liked this idea very much. Her response suggested to me that she felt neglected by Glenn.

I also suggested to Kathy that while she was staying with her sister, Glenn should give all of his money to her. Glenn would turn his paycheck over to Kathy each week, and she could pay the bills from her sister's house. If Wendy needed money from her father, he would have to tell her that he had given all of it to her mother. Kathy really approved of this idea. Glenn's giving Kathy the money would give her back some power. It would put her in a superior position to Wendy, and I hoped this would allow her to move back home, with her having some authority.

Amazingly, Glenn agreed to all of these suggestions. The partners had secret dates and Glenn turned his paycheck over to Kathy. As predicted, Glenn's giving his money to his wife infuriated his daughter. Glenn and Wendy came in to the next session together in the middle of a major fight. This was the first time I had seen the father and daughter in an argument, and they were fighting more like a husband and wife than like a parent and child. They were exchanging insults and acting as if they had both been betrayed in some way. The truth was that they had betrayed each other. Glenn had stepped over to Kathy's side, and this was a betrayal of Wendy. On the other hand, Wendy was no longer Daddy's cute girl, but was defying him, and this was a betrayal of Glenn. The issue was that Wendy had smoked marijuana again and Glenn insisted that she be grounded for the next week. I supported Glenn's decision and spent most of the session restraining him from arguing with Wendy. Afterward, when I was driving home, I wondered when I would be getting the call that Glenn and Wendy had gone home, destroyed the house, and killed each other.

To my great relief, there was no fight. Glenn stuck to his position, and he and Wendy survived until the next session. Glenn's standing up to Wendy resulted in Kathy's deciding to come home. However, she and her sister decided it would be better for their mother not to move back with Kathy and Glenn, but to stay with the sister. I thought to myself, this is one unspoken issue between Glenn and Kathy that seems to have been resolved.

The next few weeks were quiet, and I was hoping that the situation had improved. Then I received a call from Glenn. He told me that Kathy had attempted suicide. I called an emergency session and had them come in together. Kathy looked terrible. She said she had taken too many sleeping pills. She denied being suicidal, and insisted that her taking the extra pills was not an attempt to kill herself. She explained that she took Xanex at night to help her sleep, and had been doing this ever since Wendy had come home from the hospital. Having Wendy in the house made her extremely anxious. She never knew what to expect, and if she did not take the medicine, she would be up all night worrying about what Wendy might do. This was all news to me. Two nights earlier, Wendy had stayed out late again and Glenn did nothing. Kathy was so upset about this that she thought she would have to take extra pills to help her sleep. She did not take a lethal dose, but it did make her very drowsy, and this frightened Glenn.

I took this episode to mean that I still had not succeeded in breaking up the coalition between Glenn and Wendy. With Kathy out of the house, Glenn was attentive to Kathy and setting limits on Wendy. With Kathy back in the house, the old pattern had returned. Glenn was not demonstratively affectionate with his wife in the presence of his daughter, nor did he get upset with his daughter in the presence of his wife. It was the familiar problem of the man's changing when his wife threatens to leave him, but changing right back when she drops her threat.

I decided to use this pill-taking episode to go for a major change in the family. I got Glenn alone and told him that I feared that Kathy was minimizing how upset she was and that she could have accidentally harmed herself. Glenn was very shaken. I considered that a good sign and an opportunity to motivate him to change. I told him that Wendy no longer was my patient; Kathy was. I was far more concerned about her than about their daughter. I went on to say that he was going to be my co-therapist in helping his wife. This would mean he would have to go out of his way to show her how much he loved her and how devastated he would be if anything were ever to happen to her. He would have to start by telling her, before our session was over, that he loved her and did not want any harm to come to her. Glenn was desperate and easily agreed to all of this.

I then brought Kathy into the room. Glenn took her hand and told her very sincerely that he loved her and did not want her to hurt herself. Kathy was very moved, and reassured him that that was not her intent. My thought was that if I could not break up the Glenn/Wendy coalition by putting Glenn in charge of his daughter, I could break it up by putting him in charge of his wife.

The next few weeks were astounding. Glenn went all out (for him) to connect with Kathy. He sent flowers to her at her work. He took her out to dinner, something he never did. Wendy was mystified. At one point, the family came in together, and in the middle of the session, Kathy blurted out with a big grin on her face, "Glenn and I are having sex. We are keeping Wendy up at night because our bed is banging against the wall!" So much for the Glenn not being demonstrative with Kathy problem! I suggested that they put a sign on their bedroom door saying, "Do not enter, we might be having sex." The couple laughed. Wendy was mortified. For at least that one moment, I had spouses who were connected to each other and a daughter who was put in her place.

Glenn then announced that in a few weeks he was going to take Kathy to Niagara Falls for a summer vacation. They had never had a honeymoon. He had already planned the trip. Kathy was pleased. As the time approached, however, Kathy became more and more nervous about leaving Wendy at home, fearing that she might get into trouble. Wendy was still being used as a regulator of the emotional distance between the spouses. One possibility was that Kathy was reluctant to get closer to Glenn. My fear, however, was that Glenn was getting cold feet. I took the position that to allow Wendy to imprison the parents at home and prevent them from having a honeymoon was a greater problem than any trouble she might create in their absence. I put it on Glenn to reassure Kathy and insist that they go no matter what trouble Wendy might cause before their departure.

Wendy behaved and the couple went on their trip. This ended up being a major turning point. After their return, the remainder of the summer was uneventful. When school began, Kathy came in and expressed concern about Wendy's going back into the special class for kids with behavioral problems. She said she thought Wendy was much better and did not need to be in a special class, and she was worried about the possible consequences of Wendy's being labeled as difficult by the school system. I assured her that it was her right as a parent not to sign the agreement with the school that would place Wendy in the special class. I also suggested that she call the school principal, explain her concern, and offer to come to school every day, if necessary, to help settle Wendy down in regular classes. Kathy carried out this plan and the school agreed. Wendy started school in regular classes without incident.

A few months later, I had another call from Kathy. Thanksgiving was approaching and she wanted to invite Glenn's parents. This would be the first time his parents had been to the house since the trouble with Wendy began. I had Kathy and Glenn in, and we discussed their fears about how Wendy might be difficult and what they could do to prevent trouble. Glenn's parents accepted the invitation for Thanksgiving. Wendy stayed in her room most of the evening; came down for dinner, which she ate quietly at the table with the family; and then retreated to her room again afterward. The evening ended with Glenn's parents agreeing to come back. We all decided that that might be the best we could expect from Wendy, and that it could have been much worse.

Wendy had settled down, she was attending regular classes, she and her mother were getting along, Kathy and Glenn were more connected as husband and wife, his parents were associating with the family, and Kathy had found an acceptable alternative living arrangement for her mother. There was no longer any need for Wendy to be in charge.

Discussion

This case offers an example of the various roles a man can play in a family that includes a difficult adolescent. When faced with an out-of-control son or daughter and a mother who is caught up in a hostile relationship with that son or daughter, a man has two basic ways in which he can try to be helpful. He can jump into the fight and gang up on the kid, or relieve the mother in the battle. This occasionally may be effective, but my experience as a therapist with fathers who use this approach is that often it does not help. Typically, a father who reacts in this way is in a coalition with the child, and so sides with the child until the situation gets so out of hand that he must finally side with his wife.

A second way in which a father can be helpful in this situation is to involve himself with his wife. When faced with his wife and child in a hostile fight, the father can help by getting his wife out of the battle, helping her regain her composure and then dealing with the youth. He can take his wife for a walk, or up to their room, and help her to calm down. The spouses can then decide together how they want to handle their teenager. This scenario puts the father in the role of helping the mother decide how she wants to parent, as opposed to replacing the mother as the parent dealing with the child. With families in which the mother is in charge of the parenting, the helping-the-mother role allows the father to take an active part in dealing with a problem youth without overturning a hierarchical arrangement. It also gives the father something to do that clearly places him in league with the mother, undoing any implicit coalition he is in with the child. Having him go behind closed doors or for a walk with his wife is asking him to have a secret conversation with her, instead of having secret conversations with his son or daughter.

7

Men Who Vanish After Divorce or Remarriage

Divorced Dads

Fathers who vanish after a divorce are a national problem (Blankenhorn, 1995; Furstenberg & Nord, 1985; Furstenberg et al., 1987; Seltzer, 1991). These studies show that between 30% and 50% of all divorced fathers are absent. Moreover, paternal contact with the children declines over time after the divorce. In summarizing the studies reporting diminished visitation, Furstenberg stated: "Almost half of the children from recently separated couples saw their fathers once a month and one-third had not seen them at all in the past year. Among children of marriages disrupted for ten or more years, only one in ten had weekly contact with their fathers, and almost two-thirds had no contact in the past year. Over time, the vast majority of children will have little or no contact with their fathers" (Furstenberg & Cherlin, 1991, pp. 35 & 36). Hetherington (1985) found that fewer than one quarter of noncustodial fathers were seeing their children once a month after six years of divorce.

Many authors have documented the importance of a father's staying involved with his children after a divorce, and the consequences for the children when this does not happen (Hetherington, 1982, 1989; Wallerstein & Kelly, 1980a, 1980b). Sadly, despite their need for a father's vital contribution, many children lose their fathers after a divorce. Why is this happening? Perhaps the story of a divorced couple can help to shed some light on this.

Lora and Dennis married young to escape problems in their respective families. Lora had been in an especially bad situation. She did not love Dennis, but he provided a way out of her family. After the couple were married, Lora began to regret her decision but made an effort to make the marriage work. She and Dennis had two daughters together. The couple moved far away from their respective families and raised the girls with minimal involvement from the extended families. But despite her efforts, the couple had many serious problems, and after 15 years of marriage, Lora decided that she had enough. She filed for divorce. Her parents were against her decision, citing the financial difficulties she would face if she were on her own. Dennis was also against the divorce, but unwilling to make any changes that might help to salvage the marriage. He, too, had been unhappy over the years but viewed Lora as some sort of trophy that he was proud to possess. It was a blow to his self-esteem to lose her, despite the fact that he was unhappy with her, and had made few efforts over the years to better the situation. The divorce proceeded with the partners continuing to reside together, and when it was final, per the terms of the divorce, Dennis was to move out.

On the day he was to leave, however, the sparks began to fly. Privately, he had been sharing his own version of what was happening with the two girls. He had won their sympathy. When it was time for him to leave, he became very upset, cried and pleaded with Lora not to make him move. The girls were present and they also were crying and begging their mother not to split up the family. With no support from her parents, and facing her two girls begging her to change her mind, Lora backed down. The couple had an apartment above their garage, and Lora agreed to allow Dennis to live in the garage apartment.

Divorce takes place on many levels: legally, financially, geographically, sexually, emotionally, and spiritually. Confusion can result when couples divorce on some of these levels, but not on others. Lora ended up divorcing Dennis legally, sexually, emotionally, and spiritually, but stayed connected with him geographically and financially. This prevented the family from making the transition to coparenting from two separate households. It also blocked their freedom to find and develop new intimate relationships. This was, of course, what Dennis wanted.

Lora was even more miserable in this new arrangement. She wanted to move on in her life, but felt trapped. To appease her girls, she felt she had to sacrifice her need to find someone else and start a new life. She was able to sustain this sacrifice for two years. Then she met Michael, with whom she fell in love. This changed everything. The daughters were two years older and she hoped that by now they could accept the reality of what had happened between her and their father. Her new relationship also provided her with a companion who could support her decision to divorce Dennis completely. Previously, she had endured the situation all alone, with no support from anyone.

She explained to Dennis and their daughters that the family's living arrangements were going to have to end. She and Michael were planning to marry. In an attempt to block Lora's plans, Dennis again reacted by lobbying the girls. He told them that their mother cared more about Michael than about any of them, and that who knows what she and Michael might do. They might just move far away and totally abandon all of them. Dennis was dependent on and clinging to Lora. He was vulnerable, and the girls sensed this. He was using them as pawns in his quest to keep their mother. They were completely taken in. In addition to using the girls, he began to fight Lora on every conceivable financial item in the final split-up. He became very hostile, and was prone to having fits. Lora began to realize that the divorce was going to require putting some real geographical distance between herself and Dennis. She was unaware, however, of the extent to which the girls had been taken in by their father's brainwashing.

Assuming that both daughters would move with her, Lora found an apartment on the opposite side of town, in another school district. On the day that she moved, the girls informed her that they would not be joining her. She was being mean to their father, and they had no intention of leaving their familiar surroundings. Lora was crushed. She knew, however, that she could no longer tolerate the old arrangement. It was the hardest decision of her life, but she did move to her apartment, leaving the girls with their father. In her absence, Dennis was free to intensify his propaganda campaign. He pointed out to his daughters that their mother had moved away from them, and he questioned her love for them. He was using the girls to punish Lora, and it was succeeding. They were uninterested in visiting their mother. When they did, they did not stay long. Lora was totally devastated.

Several months later, Lora and Michael married and bought a house. Lora's divorce from Dennis was now complete, and she had started a new life. She was a noncustodial parent. Financially, she was much better off than Dennis. She was a professional, and both she and Michael earned good incomes. Lora paid child support, but Dennis' financial situation was not as good as hers. He had just his own income. He also had a much more difficult daily life, having to juggle full-time work with parenting two teenage girls.

Although the girls did visit Lora, she did not feel that she was really a parent. She attended their school activities and she and Michael took them on family trips together. But Lora had no day-to-day influence in her daughters' lives. She was not raising them. She had been a good mother and was very connected to them. Now, at best, she was a sideline player in their development. In addition, they continued to be angry with her and kept her at arm's length emotionally. They would go through the motions of coming to see her but they did not open up to her.

Lora had a very comfortable life. But this came at the expense of her children. In Lora's mind, it was hardly a fair trade-off. She was very depressed without the children. They had shut her out, and she knew that Dennis was the cause. Their visits with her meant very little to anyone. The girls had no enthusiasm about seeing her. Even so, it was very painful for Lora to watch them go at the end of their every-other-weekend visit. At some points, she actually considered telling the girls not to visit rather than having to experience the pain of being a sidelined parent. If the girls did not come over, Lora could escape this pain. She could immerse herself in her new marriage and try to avoid the agony of her children's rejection.

It is not hard to have empathy for single, divorced mothers.

They are often worse off financially after their divorce, and face the burden of working and raising children alone. Noncustodial fathers, on the other hand, have it made. They have more money, and they have freedom from the daily chores of raising the children. Of course, as with Lora, their freedom is accompanied by the loss of the connection that comes with the day-to-day raising of children. One could argue that, when married, many fathers were not really connected to their children anyway. They worked and their wives did most of the parenting. Even with this possibility, the reality cannot be escaped that a noncustodial parent suffers a great loss of status and influence in the children's lives even if he or she maintains a visitation schedule. In addition, Dennis was not the only custodial parent who was bitter about a spouse's leaving and used the children to punish the departed parent. Some custodial mothers are guilty of this as well, reducing the noncustodial father's influence on his children still further.

How many noncustodial fathers carry out what Lora contemplated? To avoid the pain of not being able to really father their children, they immerse themselves in their new lives. Studies show that fathers experience intense emotional pain from missing their children and having to accept a smaller role in their lives (Arendell, 1995; Hetherington & Hogan, 1986) and that some stop visiting their children to avoid this pain (Arendell, 1995; Loewen, 1986, 1988).

When parents react in this way, it does not mean that they do not care about their children. It means that they care too much. They are not avoiding their children, they are avoiding the pain of not having their children. Unfortunately, when they make this choice, they and their children lose each other. Considering that they face what Lora faced, perhaps the question of why so many fathers vanish after divorce is the wrong question. Maybe the question really is: Why not vanish?

After a year of living on the opposite side of town, Lora decided that the situation no longer was tolerable. She and Michael sold their house and moved back into the children's neighborhood. By now, Dennis had remarried, and one of the girls did not get along with their stepmother. This daughter was having serious conduct problems and moved in with Lora and Michael in their new home.

Now that Lora had returned to the daughters' neighborhood, Dennis had to stop accusing her of abandoning them. Lora now could be much more involved with her daughters. But this also came at a cost. Dennis was angry at Lora and Michael for invading his territory. He began to fight Lora on every decision associated with the new arrangement. Terms of child support would have to be changed. Dennis fought this. With one of the girls behaving badly, Lora was now more responsible for dealing with her difficulties. Dennis fought Lora about every aspect of how to help the troubled daughter. According to Dennis, the daughter's problems came as a result of Lora's "abandoning" her. Both households became war zones for the fighting parents. The girls became caught up in it, each taking the side of the parent with whom she lived. As a result of all this, tension also developed between Lora and Michael. Although she was more involved with both girls, the hostilities between Lora and Dennis took a toll on her marriage and cemented the distance between Lora and the daughter who remained with Dennis.

During this period, Lora again questioned what was really best for everyone. Her new circumstances met her need to be a mother, but with obvious costs. With all the fighting between her and Dennis, sometimes Lora wondered if it might not be better to withdraw in the interest of peace for everyone. She stuck it out until both girls had graduated from high school, however. Her marriage survived, but not without damage, and there were long-term consequences with regard to her relationship with one of her daughters.

How many noncustodial fathers have to cope with this situation? Remaining involved with the children means facing intense conflict and hostility with the ex-spouse, watching the children take sides in an ongoing war, and if either remarries, upsetting the new spouse. In this book, one main theme has been men who withdraw to avoid conflict. How many noncustodial fathers do this? In the interest of peace, they withdraw. Again, they are not withdrawing from their children, but from the war with their children's mother. But again, the real problem is that the father and children end up losing each other in the process.

Withdrawing from visitations to avoid conflict with his ex-wife is by far the most often cited reason for the father's disappearance after divorce (Arendell, 1995; Dudley, 1991; Fox, 1985; Hetherington & Hogan, 1986; Koch, 1984; Kruk, 1991). One study followed 108 families for three years after divorce (Isaacs, Montalvo, & Abelsohn, 1986). They found a strong correlation between the parents' relationship and visitation by the father after divorce and problems exhibited by the children. More specifically, they found that children best adjust to divorce if their parents can communicate in a practical manner, focusing on matters related to the children. They also found that children did best when a regular and predictable visitation schedule with the noncustodial parent was established. Chronic fighting, especially at the time of visitation pickup and drop-off, was highly associated with social and behavioral problems on the part of the children. Most important, they found that of the families in which visitation dropped off or stopped, the most common cause was a continued hostile relationship between the parents. Even with parents who started out with an acceptable visitation schedule after their divorce, if hostilities persisted for more than six months, visits were either reduced or stopped. The father stopped visiting entirely in order to avoid conflict with his ex-wife. Considering the large number of fathers who are disconnected from their children after divorce, it looks as though children are losing their fathers after divorce, and that it is attributable in large part to the phenomenon reported throughout this book: to avoid conflict, some men disappear.

The decision to withdraw from conflict with his ex-spouse, or from the pain of losing the status of day-to-day parenting, is in the hands of the men who make this choice. But, as professionals who are called upon to help in these situations, we must not be confused about what motivates a man to make such a choice. The problem is not just the man; it is also the hostile relationship between the man and his ex-wife. The man is responsible for his choices, but both parents are responsible for the relationship between them. Many single mothers seek therapy for their children who are having difficulties related to a divorce. Often the fathers are minimally involved with the children or are not involved at all. Typically, the mother has little good to say about the absent father. Even so, many studies indicate that the most upsetting consequences of divorce for children include the loss of a parent, usually the father, and having to live with a parent who is chronically bitter and angry with his or her ex-spouse. In my view, it is our obligation to these children to help the parents learn to work as a team, and when possible, to reconnect these children to their absent parent.

These are no easy tasks, but studies show that the loss of contact by noncustodial fathers is far from irreversible (Aquilino, 1993; Furstenberg, 1987). First, the custodial parent must be persuaded of the benefit of cooperation. This is impossible if the custodial parent is able to bias the therapist against the noncustodial parent. If the therapist avoids this trap, one approach he or she can use to include the noncustodial parent in the therapy process is to insist on an individual session with that parent. This way, therapists can size them up for themselves. Sometimes the mother's negative views of the father prove to be correct. But when therapists actually meet the noncustodial fathers, they often discover that the men are vastly different from how their ex-wives described them.

To join with these fathers, it is best to give them the benefit of the doubt, and not assume that they are deadbeat dads enjoying their freedom from parenthood. Therapists will get further with these fathers if they approach them with the possibility in mind that they may have withdrawn from their children to avoid fighting with the children's mother, or to avoid the pain of being a part-time parent. Although this obviously is not true of all fathers, it is best to start this way with those who are willing to meet with a therapist. The father can be asked, "What kind of relationship would you like to have with your children?"

When therapists take these steps, they discover that many divorced fathers want better relationships with their children, but do not know how to handle the hostilities with their ex-wives, or they are convinced that as noncustodial parents, they do not have much to offer. When a father describes these types of impediments to staying connected to his children, the therapist can attempt to persuade both the mother and the father that the father's involvement with their children is vital for the children. As experts, therapists can take the position with mothers and fathers that it is in the best interests of the children for both parents to learn to work together, and that fathers must be willing to stay involved even though it may be painful.

A Remarried Dad Caught Between His New Wife and His Son

Fathers who manage to stay connected to their children through the conflict of divorce and its aftermath face a new trial if they remarry. They must find a way to stay close to their children while establishing a new family and household. Some fathers find themselves caught between their new wives and their children. Conflict with their new wives over their children's visits becomes yet another cause for noncustodial fathers to discontinue visitation (Arendell, 1995). For the invisible man, a new marriage presents a whole new set of relationships to be caught between and about which to be ambivalent. One aspect of the problem seems to be the question of which household to emphasize. Once a divorced father with children is remarried, he must juggle how to divide both himself and his resources between those children and his new family. If he has children with his new wife, or if his new wife has her own children, should he emphasize his new family? After all, his new family represents the household in which he is actually living and to which he devotes most of his time. Or should he emphasize his children from his first marriage? Even though his influence with them may be greatly reduced if they do not live with him, these are his biological children. Or should he try to emphasize both households equally? I do not pretend to have the answers to these questions, nor do I think our culture has them worked out either. How fathers handle this dilemma can lead to problems in their new marriages, and/or in their relationships with their children, especially if they just try to avoid the issue.

Samuel and Tina were divorced and both had remarried. They had two sons, Jonathan, age 15, and Kevin, age 17, both of whom lived with their mother and visited their father. Samuel paid child support and stayed involved with both of the boys, until conflict with his new wife, Carrie, developed. Carrie had an 18-year-old son of her own. Her first husband did not interact with his son, and managed to pay minimal support, or none at all.

Carrie did not get along with Samuel's older son, Kevin. She felt he was disrespectful toward her. Sometimes they fought, and when they did, Carrie did not feel supported by Samuel. Tension during visits increased, culminating in a blow-up. Samuel was not home when Carrie and Kevin got into an argument that escalated. The argument ended with Kevin's punching a hole in the hallway wall and storming out of the house.

When Samuel came home, Carrie told him she would leave unless he barred Kevin from the house in the future. Samuel did not want his son's visits to end, but was afraid of losing his second wife over the issue. He capitulated. Like all invisible men, he did not agree, but he did not insist on some sort of compromise. He just went along with Carrie's demand. A cold war ensued between Kevin and Carrie. Kevin was told that he was not to visit, and he gladly complied in an attempt to punish his father for taking Carrie's side. Samuel then began a secret relationship with Kevin; he would meet him for lunch and not inform Carrie that he was doing so. Samuel was so afraid of Carrie's threat of leaving that he could not admit to her that he was having a relationship with his son outside the home. This continued for several months, until the holidays arrived.

As Thanksgiving approached, Samuel begged Carrie to allow Kevin to attend the family dinner. With trepidation, Carrie relented, but only under the condition that Kevin apologize to her for the angry incident. This sounded reasonable, but it was a big request. It implied that Kevin was responsible for the problems, and this did not match how he and his father were assessing the situation in their secret meetings. Samuel was not setting limits with either Carrie or Kevin. He was just patronizing both. When Samuel explained to Kevin that he would have to apologize to

Carrie if he were to join them for Thanksgiving, Kevin felt betrayed. Finally, giving in to his father's pleading, Kevin swallowed his pride and apologized to his stepmother, but it did not make for a happy visit. Kevin ate Thanksgiving dinner with them, but the scene was very tense.

After the holidays, Kevin visited his father's home only infrequently. He and his father continued their private meetings, however. This went on until Kevin graduated from high school.

By the time Kevin was ready for his freshman year in college, Carrie's son was entering his second year at a local university. Samuel was helping to pay Carrie's son's tuition, and he was stretched thin financially. With both boys in college, Carrie's son would have to take out larger loans, and perhaps transfer to a less expensive school. Carrie erupted. She wanted the family resources devoted to her son, not to the belligerent Kevin. She was advocating for her child. This was understandable, but Samuel was not advocating for his son. Again, rather than demand some sort of compromise, Samuel backed down and agreed to the arrangement he and Carrie already had set up whereby he would contribute to Carrie's son's tuition. He allowed his new wife to interfere in his relationship with his son. Rather than insist that his sons, and his financial responsibility to them, came with him when he married Carrie, he agreed to a situation in which the emphasis would be placed on supporting his stepson and his new household at the expense of his obligations to his own sons.

Although he had initially agreed to help pay for his son's tuition, when it came time to send the payment, he said he could not afford it. He blamed his financial difficulties on having to pay both child support for his younger son and college tuition for Kevin. Kevin was furious and deeply disappointed in his father. He was forced to take additional loans and to attend a less expensive school than planned. In Kevin's mind, he essentially had lost his father.

Samuel was not willing to advocate for his son in view of Carrie's threats of divorce. Not surprisingly, the relationship became problematic. Not willing to assert himself with Carrie, Samuel pretended that everything was fine between them, but found every excuse he could to keep her at a distance. He worked long hours. He withdrew from her emotionally and sexually, but did not admit that he was disturbed. Carrie began to feel neglected and feared that Samuel was not being honest with her. It did not occur to her that he was angry with her for putting him in such a difficult position with his son. She assumed, because verbally Samuel always went along with her, that Samuel was just as mad at Kevin as she was. She knew that something was wrong, but did not know what. Finally, she sought help.

When Samuel and Carrie came to my office, Samuel confessed to me privately that the problem was that there was a war on between Carrie and his son Kevin. It had to be dragged out of him, but he did tell me about the college-tuition question, and that he felt he was being prevented from helping his son. With help, he was able to tell the truth to his wife. He was upset with her. He had withdrawn. It was over her conflict with Kevin. Again Carrie threatened to leave. I asked her, "Do you really want to force your husband to stop helping his own son? What would be said if the situation were reversed? What if a new husband threatened to leave his wife unless she did not associate with one of her children?"

Carrie said she knew she was wrong, but when Kevin did visit, he was very obnoxious to her, and Samuel would stand by and say nothing. Then she accused Samuel of conducting a relationship with Kevin behind her back. Apparently, she had known all along what was going on. I looked at Samuel, and he just sat there silently.

With much difficulty, a new arrangement was negotiated. Samuel agreed to stop all secret meetings with Kevin and to set limits on him when he treated Carrie disrespectfully. The hard part was getting Carrie to allow financial resources to be devoted to Kevin's college expenses. I took the position that if she really wanted to be closer to Samuel, she was going to have to agree that Samuel could help his son. Reluctantly, she went along.

Both Samuel and Carrie kept their agreements. Samuel stopped meeting Kevin in secret and managed, to Kevin's great consternation, to insist that he treat his stepmother with respect when he was at their house. He did offer financial help to Kevin, and apparently this helped the marriage. The couple reported in their last session with me that they were spending more time together. Carrie no longer felt neglected.

A Man Caught Between His Wife and His Ex-Wife

Rebecca was 27, lived with her 52-year-old mother, and was an alcoholic. She was accompanied to her first appointment with me by both of her biological parents, Ted and Andrea. Andrea had called to schedule the first appointment, and suggested that she come with her daughter and her ex-husband. After graduating from college, Rebecca had moved from job to job, was unable to sustain an independent living arrangement, and had been in and out of several relationships over the past few years. At the first session, her parents reported that they feared she had a serious drinking problem. She had incurred several charges of driving while intoxicated over the past several years, and admitted to being a binge drinker. Although both of her parents were very concerned about her, Rebecca minimized her drinking and stated that she could quit if she wanted to. She only came to the initial appointment at her mother's insistence.

Andrea and Ted had been divorced for almost 10 years and Ted had been remarried for nine. Andrea had not married again after the divorce, but had had various relationships. At the first session, it was obvious that Andrea was obsessed with Rebecca's problems, and was dictating what should be done about them. Ted also expressed concern, but did not offer any differing opinions. He appeared to be deferring to whatever Andrea said. When asked what Ted's wife, Patricia, thought about it, and whether she had been invited to the session, a quiet came over the room. Rebecca volunteered that she did not feel very supported by Patricia and that she had not wanted Patricia to attend. When Ted was asked about it, he sat silently and offered only a feeble response.

Rebecca had been in various treatment programs over the past several years, none of which had been helpful. Andrea was looking for someone who would work with Rebecca individually, and keep Ted and her apprised of Rebecca's progress. To me, the request seemed doomed to fail. First, Rebecca did not appear to be asking for any help. Second, it looked as though Andrea had been running the show, and the way she was running it had, for whatever reason, not been effective. Third, to just summarily exclude Ted's wife from the process seemed unwise. I asked the parents to define what they would consider progress by Rebecca. They described sensible objectives, such as her finding and keeping a job that was worthy of her potential, her establishing financial independence, her not just jumping from man to man, and her controlling her drinking habit. Rebecca said she, too, would like to find a good job and attain financial independence. Although she did not think it was necessary, she also agreed to reduce her drinking. I asked how she fared financially. I got a vague answer. She was currently "rooming" with her mother, and her father helped her out by paying some of her bills from time to time. She had car payments to make and some credit card debt.

I said that I would agree to see Rebecca individually on an occasional basis if she so requested, but that the best way I could assist her would be to conduct family meetings focusing on what everyone could do to help Rebecca get on her feet. If they were interested in this, I would want Ted's wife, Patricia, to be included. Rebecca was hesitant about accepting my offer. Both parents were in favor of it, however, and when Rebecca protested, they encouraged her to give it a try.

The therapy proceeded with Rebecca, Ted, Patricia, and Andrea coming in together to try to set some goals for Rebecca and to discuss how everyone could be of help. Patricia did not seem unsupportive, contrary to Rebecca's earlier assertions. If anything, she seemed very tentative and was apologetic before offering any ideas.

Initially, Rebecca seemed to make progress, but not far into the process, she had a major binge drinking episode. Andrea found her at home passed out. She had drunk an entire bottle of vodka. Andrea took her to the hospital, where she stayed for three days to detox and be under observation.

When Rebecca was released, I brought the family together, and started over with a new plan. As the therapy went on, it became evident that Andrea, although very agreeable in the sessions, was not keeping her agreements outside of the sessions. She would make decisions for Rebecca on her own, which contradicted what we agreed to in our sessions. I asked Andrea to meet with me alone to make sure I was not missing something. She insisted that I was not. She said that during the period between sessions, she would just get an idea about what to do and go with it. She was not dissatisfied with our planning during the sessions. Andrea's impulsive decision making was undermining my attempts to organize a unified plan among all of the participants, but it was clear that she was in charge and that if I lost her, I would lose the case. I gently appealed to her to make sure to let me know if I suggested something, or if the group came up with something, with which she did not agree. She cheerfully accepted my proposal.

The therapy continued, and despite the fact that all were attending and seemed to be agreeing on a course of action, Rebecca continued to have binge drinking episodes. I was confused by the fact that even though everyone seemed to reach agreements in my office, Rebecca continued to struggle. I felt there was something very important that I still did not know that would explain the situation. I was concerned that Andrea was stuck in her life, not able to move on after her divorce from Ted, and that Rebecca's problems helped to organize her. I did not feel it was proper to bring this up with Rebecca continuing to struggle, however. I assumed that if Rebecca could sustain an improvement, Andrea's problems would become apparent. Otherwise, I thought the focus of the therapy had to be on Rebecca.

At one point, both Andrea and Rebecca began to push the idea that Rebecca needed to find her own apartment. Andrea was nervous about finding Rebecca drunk on the couch again, and no longer was comfortable living with her. I did not think this was a good idea. First, it had become clear that Rebecca was in a pattern of moving out on her own and then relapsing back to living with Andrea. This seemed like a repetition of that pattern. Second, Rebecca had not made sufficient progress to be able to maintain an independent living arrangement. I advised that she stay with her mother until she had improved enough to inspire confidence that she could make it on her own. Andrea reluctantly agreed, but I feared the therapy was in trouble.

The next week, I got a call from Ted and Patricia requesting that just the two of them come to see me. I met with them privately, and they enlightened me on the mystery. Since my last meeting with the family, Andrea had decided that despite Rebecca's continuing to struggle, she was going to have to move out. However, Rebecca had only a part-time job as a waitress. She had no money saved and could not maintain her own apartment without help. Although Andrea was a professional, she could not afford to support both herself and Rebecca. She called Ted and persuaded him to set Rebecca up in her own apartment. Without discussing the idea with his wife, Ted agreed that if Andrea and Rebecca could find an apartment within a certain price range, he would pay the first month's rent. After that, he expected Rebecca to pay her own way. She did find an apartment, but the rent was several hundred dollars per month more than what Ted had agreed to pay.

Ted thought he was being firm by agreeing to pay only the first month's rent. Patricia was silent, however. I asked why they had wanted to tell me this in private. Patricia finally spoke. She said that over the past nine years, Ted had given thousands of dollars to Andrea to help Rebecca. This was the fourth or fifth apartment he had financed. He had also bought Rebecca cars, which she had totaled, and paid for treatment for Rebecca that Andrea had arranged without consulting anyone. With this latest episode, Patricia said she was happy that Ted was setting a one-month limit, but based on his past behavior, she had little confidence that he would be able to stick to it.

Ted looked at me and asked, "What am I supposed to do, let my daughter become homeless?" I asked Patricia if her not being consulted about Ted's helping financially was also part of the pattern. Patricia broke into tears. She said she had been labeled the "evil stepmother" because she had protested in the past about continuing to offer money when it had not proved to be helpful. She said she had never been consulted, but just informed that another round of financial assistance had begun. She felt as though

Ted's ex-wife were in charge of his finances. She and Ted had had to sacrifice trips in the past because Ted had agreed to devote the money to helping Rebecca. Patricia said she was not opposed to Ted's helping his daughter, but that she was totally excluded from the decisions, and it had long been clear that he was just throwing the money away. This latest episode had pushed Patricia to the brink. She said that if it did not stop, she was through.

I looked at Ted and asked, "Why are you doing this?" He said that Andrea had always called him at his office and could get him to agree to anything. He was not able to say "No" to her. He could not do it when they were married, and he could not do it after they divorced. He knew it was taking a toll on his present marriage, but he did not realize how much. Patricia was not asking Ted not to help his daughter, she was asking to be included in the decisions. Andrea had managed to keep a secret relationship with Ted regarding parenting Rebecca. In this sense, Ted and Andrea had never divorced. By committing money to Andrea and Rebecca behind his wife's back, Ted was not standing up for his second marriage. To keep peace with his daughter and his ex-wife, he was giving them the money they requested against his better judgment. He was caught between his wife and his ex-wife, and he was handling it by being invisible. He said he had always felt guilty about leaving Andrea and Rebecca, and he felt obligated to give them what they asked. He did not want it to cost him his new marriage, however.

I was in a bind. On the one hand, Patricia had come in and clearly stated that she could not stay in her marriage as it was. She had never said this before. On the other hand, any advice I gave the couple in the absence of Andrea would surely lead to Andrea's firing me. As I pondered the situation, I wondered who my client was. It was clear from the start that it was not Rebecca. She only came because her parents had dragged her in and she was not changing in any meaningful way. I had originally thought that Andrea was my client, but she never stuck to her agreements and just went about doing what she wanted to do, disregarding any plan to which she may have agreed in the sessions. The latest apartment episode was just another example. It seemed clear that until this session, no one was really requesting help to change. Rebecca had no reason to change. She was getting whatever she wanted. Andrea seemed genuinely concerned about Rebecca, but was not willing to follow any suggestions that deviated from whatever she wanted to do. In this session, however, Patricia and Ted were clearly asking for help. I decided to go with that.

I suggested to Ted that to save his marriage he was going to have to change how he was handling the situation. He agreed. I took the position that it was not clear whether or not offering more financial help at this time was a good idea, but that whatever the decision would be, Patricia should be included in it. Since any financial help would essentially come from both Ted and Patricia, it was my advice that no money be offered unless both Ted and Patricia participated in the decision. Patricia was very appreciative of this idea and Ted said he knew it was the right thing to do. He said it would result in agitating both Andrea and Rebecca, however. I said that all he would be asking would be that his marriage of 10 years be respected. That did not mean he was cutting his daughter off. He said he realized this. I suggested we invite Andrea in and Ted could explain his decision with my help. The session ended with a plan for Ted to come back with Andrea and describe the process he wanted to establish for making future decisions regarding financial help for Rebecca.

A week later, I found a long message from Andrea on my answering machine. She was very polite. She said she thought I had been helpful, but that she did not need to come back for any future sessions. I then received a call from Ted. He reported that he had decided to tell Andrea of his decision on his own. He said she listened politely, but he feared the worst. Patricia, on the other hand, was very happy with him. Rebecca was not. He had decided to set a limit on the amount he would give her. This was the first time he had ever done this. No additional appointments were scheduled.

I followed up with Patricia several months later. Ted had indeed stuck to his position. Not only did he limit how much money he gave Rebecca for her apartment, but he also blocked a subsequent attempt by Andrea to secretly get him to give more. He talked to Patricia before responding. Rebecca had moved back with her mother. Ted had saved his marriage, however, and was finally acting as though he was more married to Patricia than to his ex-wife.

Helping a Stepfather Have a Presence

It has been the conventional wisdom in our field that new stepparents should ease their way into a parenting role with their stepchildren. The idea is that stepparents should start by establishing a positive relationship with the children before attempting to participate in their discipline. This advice seems reasonable, but if a stepparent is going to be integrated into the family, especially if the stepparent and children are under the same roof, he or she is going to have to assume a role that is consistent with the day-to-day responsibilities of raising children. For a stepfather, assuming his wife wants him to act as a parent to the children, this means eventually asserting his authority. To be a parent, it is not enough to have a loving relationship with children. Sometimes a parent has to intervene and set limits. This is hard enough for some biological fathers, and is especially difficult for a man who is not really the children's father. This seems like just the setup for some men to disappear.

Jonathan and Erica had been married for six years and had three children of their own. Erica had been married before and had one son, David. After being divorced from David's father for three years, Erica married Jonathan. At the time, David was 6 years old and living with his mother. David's father stayed involved with him after the divorce, and when Jonathan and Erica were married, he did not interfere with Jonathan's establishing a relationship with David. Jonathan worked hard at connecting with David. He took him fishing and to the movies, and made a point of establishing a positive relationship with the boy. He was very careful not to put David in a loyalty bind between himself and David's father, and insisted that David call him Jonathan. Despite Jonathan's efforts, and the collaboration of all of the adults, by the time David was a teenager, he had developed some behavior problems and the family sought help from me.

Jonathan, Erica, and David came to the first session without the rest of their children. They gave the history, and I said they were to be congratulated for being so careful about seeing that Jonathan and David got connected. After several sessions, we were still struggling to make progress, and it was unclear why. The typical pattern of the biological parent's blocking the stepparent's attempts to parent did not seem to be evident. The two parents seemed to be in agreement on how to deal with David's difficulties. David's father did not seem to be a problem either. He had stayed involved, but appeared to be supportive of Erica and Jonathan's efforts. The adults seemed sufficiently organized to settle the boy down and did not appear to be undermining each other. This was confirmed by the way in which the parents responded to suggestions for getting David to calm down. They collaborated with one another and I was confused as to why their efforts to work together had not solved the problem.

One thing that had not occurred in the therapy thus far was that I had not met with the entire household. Despite my requests, the three younger children had not been able to attend a session together with both parents and David. Finally, everyone came to the fourth session. In the first five minutes of the meeting, the mystery was solved. First, the family seating was revealing. Jonathan sat on the couch with the three younger children, while Erica and David sat on chairs next to each other. Then, during the session, the 2-year-old daughter became a nuisance and the knee-jerk reaction was for Jonathan to take the girl out of the room and calm her down, while Erica stayed with David in the therapy room. The family was revealing its structure, and it was very telling. A short episode involving David's being defiant gave me my final clues. Jonathan told a story of how he had asked David to take out the trash and, as usual, David erupted. Jonathan asked him again to do his chore, but David refused. Erica insisted that David do as he was told. David then reluctantly obeyed.

After the scene in the office with Jonathan and the 2-year-old, it seemed clear that Jonathan did not hesitate to deal with his three biological children when circumstances demanded it. When the 2-year-old acted up, he attempted to intervene, and when she did not respond, without hesitation, Jonathan just picked her up and took her out of the room. In their story about the trash, however, Jonathan was not so assertive. He instructed David to take out the trash, but he did not follow through when David refused. Erica had to intervene. I began to wonder whether David might not be jealous of his younger siblings. He was the only child in the home who was not Jonathan's biological child. Although Jonathan had maintained a positive relationship with David, he did not treat David as he did the other children. He did not lay down the law as he did to his own children. Only Erica did that. That put Jonathan and the three younger children in one camp and Erica and David in another. It looked to me as though David wanted his stepdad to really climb all over him if he screwed up, just as he did with the other children.

I accused Jonathan of playing favorites. He agreed. He said he did more fun things with David than with his own children. I disagreed. I pointed out that David did not have the same privileges as the other three. Both Jonathan and Erica could not imagine what those privileges might be. I said there were two privileges that the three younger children had that David did not have. First, David did not have the privilege of calling Jonathan "Dad." After all, after six years, Jonathan certainly had fathered David. He was helping to raise David on a daily basis. He had taken care of David when he fell sick. He supported the family. He gave David fatherly lessons. Jonathan was like a father, but he insisted that David call him by his first name. Jonathan said that was out of respect for David's real dad. I said I understood, but what if David wanted to call Jonathan "Dad." Jonathan said that had never occurred to him, but it was OK if David wanted to. David instantly brightened up.

Second, David did not have the privilege of getting a proper fatherly chewing out when he deserved one. The other three children certainly got it when they deserved it. Only David was left out. When he messed up, Jonathan would scold him but then let his mother come in and finish him off. Jonathan was not asserting himself when David needed him to. Instead, he was just correcting him feebly and then disappearing behind the scenes. David was being deprived of really experiencing the authority of a man. Erica instantly chimed in. She wanted Jonathan to take a stronger hand with David. I predicted that it would be hard for her to let Jonathan do so since she was so accustomed to jumping in automatically when David needed to be corrected. She agreed. We all decided that for the next two weeks, only Jonathan would get after David when he did something wrong. Erica's job when this occurred would be to look after the little ones so that Jonathan could concentrate totally on David. I asked the couple to reverse for two weeks the family structure they had established and demonstrated so clearly in my office.

In two weeks the family returned in good spirits. Jonathan had called David's father, and explained what we had been discussed. He asked him if it would be all right if David called him Dad like the other children did. David's father understood and said it was OK. David began to call Jonathan Dad, once he realized that *Jonathan* was OK with it. This made a big change in the home that did not go unnoticed by the three younger children. Once David was calling him Dad, Jonathan began to act more like one, but not without slaying some internal dragons. He had grown up without a father and so had no role model to look back to, to be either like or unlike. It was very difficult for him to bring himself to assert his authority for the first time. Several opportunities passed before, finally, David screwed up and Jonathan got after him as planned. Erica had no problem with it, and David actually seemed pleased. One month later, the family returned and assumed a new seating arrangement. Both parents sat together and the four children sat on the couch. I took this to indicate that a significant structural shift had taken place, and I felt the therapy was over. Coincidentally, David's behavior had also improved.

8

Evaluating Power in Relationships

Two young children, a brother and a sister, lived with their father and stepmother. The father was prominent in his community. His first wife, the children's mother, had died and he had remarried, partly to find a mother for his children. He had many responsibilities and basically turned his children over to his new wife for her to raise. She found herself in a situation in which she had the responsibility of raising children whom she barely knew with minimal help from her husband. We can assume that she must have become very resentful about this. She began to treat the children badly. She abused them, both verbally and physically. The father was aware of her treatment of his children, but he did not intervene. He feared the anger of his new wife and so did not advocate for better treatment of his children. Like many of the men described in this book, he allowed his wife to dominate him with the threat of becoming angry. Rather than asserting himself, he withdrew. The abuse of the children continued, and finally, knowing their father was not going to protect them, they ran away from home. At this point, their story took a tragic turn. After running away, they wandered around their neighborhood and eventually were taken in by what they thought was a kindly old woman. They were never seen or heard from again.

A second story also concerns a husband and his second wife. Again, this man's first wife had died. The couple had had one child, a daughter. The man was also prominent in his community, and did not remarry for many years. He and his daughter became very close, and by the time he remarried, his daughter was in her middle to late teens. His new wife became very aware of how fond the man was of his daughter, and she became jealous. When around his daughter, the father displayed his affection for her. He was not as generous with his affections to his new wife. Of course, when directly confronted by his wife with the question of whether he found her attractive, he said all the right things. He patronized her. The wife was in a situation in which her husband said one thing, but did another. She became very insecure and obsessed with the question of whom her husband was more fond, her or his daughter. The wife was so concerned about this question that she would stand in front of her mirror daily and compare herself physically with her stepdaughter. Not surprisingly, powerful hostilities developed between the stepmother and stepdaughter. Again, as with the other men in this book, the father did not intervene between his wife and daughter. His silence conveyed tolerance for the problems, and so perpetuated them. The hostilities between the stepmother and the stepdaughter continued until, finally, the daughter was forced to leave the family. The legend of this family grew in the community and focused on the cruelty and insecurities of the stepmother. As usual, everyone missed the contribution of the father, who was patronizing toward his wife, silent when the problems developed, and confused about what he should do.

These two stories fit right in with the cases we have been examining and so by now should be very familiar. The interesting thing is that they are both centuries old and come from a time when their respective societies were legally very patriarchal. The first story is that of Hansel and Gretel, and the second story is that of Snow White. It seems there is the possibility that the patterns we have been examining in this book have been around for ages. It is interesting that even though the stories come from a time in which women could not own property and otherwise were discriminated against legally, we could read about such families and take it for granted that the men in the stories were weak and dominated by their wives.

Another, more recent, story also represents women as powerful and men as weak. This is the story of a teenage girl who lived with her parents on a farm in the American Midwest during the 1930s. She was a strong-willed, energetic girl who was not afraid to assert herself and was not afraid to challenge the powerful upper class in her county. Her mother no doubt was her role model. Although the mother performed the typical duties of a wife on a farm, such as cooking meals for all of the farm hands, she was clearly in charge. She kept a close watch on the farm hands and did not hesitate to assert herself with them and give them orders.

The girl had a pet dog of which she was very fond and that followed her everywhere. But every day on her way home from school, when the girl passed by a very prominent woman's property, her dog would harass the woman. This was a very wealthy, powerful woman who was known for being mean-spirited. Finally, after several nasty encounters between the woman and the dog, the woman came to the farm and demanded that the dog be put to sleep. The girl, of course, was taken aback and became very upset. She first pleaded with her father not to let the woman take her dog. The father just shook his head, sat down, and looked over at his wife, as if deferring to her to decide how to handle it. The wife was beside herself, but feared the power of the woman. She decided that her daughter's dog would have to go.

An interesting thing about this scene is that when faced with a crucial decision, one of those defining moments when power is revealed, the woman of the house made the decision and her husband deferred to her. In this case, the parents of the girl were not really her parents, they were her aunt and uncle. The story is "The Wizard of Oz." Again, we have an example of a story that takes place during a time when men were thought of as dominant and women were thought of as passive, yet within the family, it was Aunt Em who had the power.

Haley also provides data that throw into question how power is distributed within a family (Haley, 1996). He was conducting research on families in the 1950s. One of the goals of the research was to have families allow themselves to be observed while performing a task or having a structured conversation. In one group, the families had adolescents who had been diagnosed as psychotic or delinquent. A second group of families had adolescents with no diagnoses. At one point, Haley became interested in how the second group of families had made the decision to participate in the research. He checked a sample of 30 of these families.

In 27 out of the 30 families, when originally called by the research project's recruiter, the mother answered the phone. When asked if her family might be interested in participating, the mother answered Yes. She did not say, "I'll have to consult my husband." She made a unilateral decision. All 27 of these families participated in the research project. The mother had the power to get her family to come, apparently without consulting anyone. In two of the 30 families, the father answered the original recruitment call. In these two instances, the father said his family would participate. The fathers made this decision on the phone, without consulting their wives. These two families did not show up for the research project. In the last family, the husband answered the recruitment call, and when asked if his family would participate, he said he would have to consult his wife. This family did participate.

Clearly, power within particular relationships is not a simple thing to determine. How a couple verbally describes who is in charge within the relationship does not seem to be a predictor of how power is distributed within that relationship. Social anthropologists have long known that within a given group, or tribe, a family member who is said to have power is often not the one who actually has it (Kuper, 1996). A society can be "patriarchal" and "male dominated," yet with a particular couple, the wife can be dominant. To understand a particular couple, a therapist must have no prior bias and the couple's behavior must be directly observed to determine who actually decides what will be done in a given circumstance.

The pattern we have been observing is one in which one partner has a fear of angering, or upsetting, the other, and so capitulates to the partner's demands without negotiating. The capitulating partner withdraws or patronizes. He or she does not assert himself or herself. This then creates a power imbalance, with the capitulating spouse one down. Some women face this situation, for example, women in relationships in which domestic violence is occurring. Fearing that she might be battered, the woman capitulates on any issue that may anger her husband. Presumably, the pattern of one partner's capitulating to the other to avoid the partner's anger can be seen in any long-term relationship between two individuals. This book is about men who are the ones in relationships who are afraid to upset their spouse and so capitulate.

When a power imbalance does exist between partners, it renders the possibility of fair negotiations impossible. There will then be pressure to equalize power, if not by direct means, then indirectly. Obviously, either member of any long-term dyad can be faced with a power imbalance in the relationship. Invariably, therapists working with couples, or individuals, can be drawn into aligning with women they determine to be one down in the relationship. It is difficult not to side with the underdog. The problem, as has been discussed in earlier chapters, is that the one with whom a therapist decides to align in a problem relationship can either change, or reinforce, the couple's unfortunate patterns. I have argued in this book that to help a couple change when one partner is apparently one down, the task is to get the one-down partner to elevate himself or herself. The first step is to accurately determine who is in the one-down position. That means understanding power in relationships.

Haley argued that many relationships can be understood by assuming a dual power structure, an unofficial one and an official one (Haley, 1996). Thinking in stereotypes, this concept is easily demonstrated. One stereotype is the male boss and his female secretary. Officially, the boss is the head of the company. He is the bottom line and he earns the salary to prove it. But his secretary is in charge of his schedule. She determines what he will do every day, whom he will meet with, and how long the meeting will take. She organizes him. This is a lot of power. Unofficially, she is in charge of the day-to-day activities of her boss. But she does not have the authority, or get the credit or the salary proportional to this responsibility. A dual hierarchy exists in which the boss has official power and the secretary has unofficial power. Their status is different, but their power differential is not what it appears to be.

The doctor and the nurse provide another example. Officially, the doctor is in charge of making treatment decisions and earns the salary defining higher status. Unofficially, especially in psychiatry, the nurse is the one who spends the most time with the patient and is the one to whom the patient opens up. For these reasons, the nurse is often much more knowledgeable than the doctor about how to help a particular patient. The doctor may become reliant on the nurse's advice and knowledge to make treatment decisions. Unofficially, the nurse has power. But again, the nurse does not have the authority, or the salary, or get the credit that goes along with that responsibility. A dual hierarchy exists that blurs power, but again, status is clearly different.

Looking at these stereotypes, and the fairy tales and other anecdotal stories, we come back to Jackson (1965), who argued that power is always equal in long-term dyads. As my colleague Neil Schiff describes it, couples agree on how to be unequal. I would add that status may be different, but power is equal. Therapists intervening in these dyads would be wise to keep this idea in mind before aligning, purposefully or inadvertently, with one spouse or the other. This would seem to be especially relevant when working with a family in which a man has disappeared. He may have status, but just be a figurehead. In a society that continues to struggle with equality between the sexes *outside* of the family, *within* some families, a man can find himself one down. In these instances, instead of equalizing the relationship in an overt way by asserting himself, he may use a covert method and withdraw and become invisible. To get an invisible man to appear and make his presence felt, he, not the wife, must be elevated from a one-down position. What I have found is that within these families, the woman knows that the man is struggling, and is giving up his overt influence. When this happens, often the woman is grateful when a therapist helps the man to assert himself and become overtly involved as an equal partner.

References

Agulink, P. (1970). The spouse of the phobic patient. *Archives of General Psychiatry, 117*, 59–67.

Aquilino, W. (1993). Impact of childhood family structure and later-life parental divorce on young adults' relationship with parents. Unpublished manuscript, University of Wisconsin–Madison, Department of Child and Family Studies.

Arendell, T. (1995). *Fathers and divorce*. London: Sage.

Barlow, D., & O'Brien, G. (1984). Couples treatment of agoraphobia. *Behavior Therapy, 15*, 41–58.

Berg, B., & Rosenblum, N. (1978). Fathers in family therapy: A survey of family therapists. *Journal of Marriage and Family Counseling, 3*, 85–91.

Biller, H. B. (1981a). The father and sex role development. In M. E. Lamb (Ed.), *The role of the father in child development*. New York: Wiley.

Biller, H. B. (1981b). Father absence, divorce and personality development. In M. E. Lamb (Ed.), *The role of the father in child development*. New York: Wiley.

Birdwhistell, R. (1970). *Kinesics and context*. Philadelphia: University of Pennsylvania Press.

Blankenhorn, D. (1995). *Fatherless America*. New York: Basic Books.

Brownell, K. (1978). The effect of couples training and partner cooperativeness in the behavioral treatment of obesity. *Behavior Research and Therapy, 16*, 323–333.

Budd, K., & O'Brien, T. (1982). Father involvement in behavioral parent training. *Journal of the American Behavior Modification Association, 5*, 85–89.

Carr, A. (1998). The inclusion of fathers in family therapy: A research based perspective. *Contemporary Family Therapy, 20*, 371–383.

Dudley, J. (1991). Increasing our understanding of divorced fathers who have infrequent contact with their children. *Family Relations, 40*, 279–285.

Erickson, M. (1980). A shocking breakout of a mother's domination. In E. Rossi (Ed.), *The collected papers of Milton H. Erickson, Vol. IV* (pp. 476–481). New York: Irvington.

Fry, W. (1962). The marital context of an anxiety syndrome. *Family Process*, Sept., 245–252.

Furstenberg, F., et al. (1987). Parental participation and children's well-being after marital dissolution. *American Sociological Review, 52*, 695–701.

Furstenberg, F., & Cherlin, A. (1991). *Divided families: What happens to children when parents part?* Cambridge, MA: Harvard University Press.

Furstenberg, F., & Nord, C. (1985). Parenting apart: Patterns of childrearing after marital disruption. *Journal of Marriage and the Family, 47*, 893–904.

Goodstein, R., & Swift, K. (1977). Psychotherapy with phobic patients: The marriage relationship as the source of symptoms and focus of treatment. *American Journal of Psychotherapy, 31*, 285–292.

Grove, D., & Haley, J. (1992). *Conversations on therapy.* New York: Norton.

Gurman, A., & Kniskern, M. (1978). Research on marital and family therapy: Progress, perspective and prospect. In S. L. Garfield (Ed.), *Handbook of psychotherapy and behavior change* (2nd ed.). New York: Wiley.

Hafner, J. (1977). The husbands of agoraphobic women and their influence on treatment outcomes. *British Journal of Psychiatry, 131*, 289–294.

Hafner, J. (1983). Agoraphobic women married to abnormally jealous men. *British Journal of Medical Psychology, 52*, 99–104.

Hafner, J., & Ross, M. (1983). Predicting the outcome of behavior therapy for agoraphobia. *Behavior Research and Therapy*, 375–382.

Haley, J. (1959). An interactional description of schizophrenia. *Psychiatry, 22* (4), 321–332.

Haley, J. (1967). Toward a theory of pathological systems. In G. Zuk (Ed.), *Family therapy and disturbed families*. Palo Alto, CA: Science & Behavior Books.

Haley, J. (1973). *Uncommon therapy*. New York: Norton.

Haley, J. (1976). *Problem solving therapy*. San Francisco: Jossey-Bass.

Haley, J. (1983). *Conversations with Milton H. Erickson. Vols. I, II, III*. New York: Triangle.

Haley, J. (1992). *Jay Haley on Milton Erickson*. New York: Brunner/Mazel.

Haley, J. (1994). Personal communication.

Haley, J. (1996). *Teaching and learning therapy*. New York: Guilford.

Haley, J. (1997). *Leaving home* (2nd ed.). New York: Brunner/Mazel.

Hall, N. (1989). *Broodmales*. Dallas: Spring Publications.

Hecker, L. (1991). Where is Dad? 21 ways to involve fathers in family therapy. *Journal of Family Psychotherapy, 2*, 31–45.

Hetherington, E. M. (1985). Long term effects of divorce and remarriage on the adjustment of children. *Journal of the American Academy of Child Psychiatry, 24*, 518–530.

Hetherington, E. M., & Hogan, M. (1986). Divorced fathers: Stress, coping and adjustment. In M. Lamb (Ed.), *The father's role: Applied perspectives*. New York: Wiley.

Hetherington, E. M., et al. (1978). The aftermath of divorce. In J. H. Stevens (Ed.), *Mother/child, father/child relationships*. Washington, DC: National Association for the Education of Young Children.

Heubeck, B. (1986). Father involvement and responsibility in family therapy. In M. E. Lamb (Ed.), *The father's role: Applied perspectives*. New York: Wiley.

Issacs, M., Montalvo, B., & Abelsohn, D. (1986). *The difficult divorce*. New York: Basic Books.

Jackson, D. (1961). International psychotherapy. *Contemporary Psychotherapies*, 256–271.

Jackson, D. (1965). Family rules. Marital quid pro quo. *Archives of General Psychiatry, 12*, 589–594.

Koch, M. (1984). Visitation and the noncustodial father. *Journal of Divorce, 8*, 47–65.

Kotelchuck, M. (1981). The infant's relationship to the father: Experimental evidence. In M. E. Lamb (Ed.), *The role of the father in child development*. New York: Wiley.

Kruk, E. (1991). Discontinuity between pre- and post-divorce father-child relationships. New evidence regarding paternal disengagement. In C. Everett (Ed.), *The consequences of divorce* (pp. 195–227). New York: Haworth.

Kuper, A. (1996). *The chosen primate*. Cambridge, MA: Harvard University Press.

La Barbera, J. D., & Lewis, S. (1980). Fathers who undermine children's treatment. *Journal of Clinical Child Psychology, 1*, 367–373.

L'Abate, L. (1975). Pathogenic role rigidity in fathers, some observations. *Journal of Marriage and Family Counseling*, 69–77.

LaFave, M. K. (1980). Correlates of engagement in family therapy. *Journal of Marital and Family Therapy, 6*, 75–81.

Lamb, M. E. (1981). *The role of the father in child development*. New York: Wiley.

Lamb, M. E. (1986). *The father's role: Applied perspectives*. New York: Wiley.

Lamb, M. E. (1989). *Fatherhood and family policy*. New York: Wiley.

Lederer, W., & Jackson, D. (1968). *The mirages of marriage*. New York: Norton.

Loewen, J. (1986). A comparison of maternal, paternal and joint custody: Understanding the varieties of postdivorce family life. *Journal of Divorce, 9*, 1–12.

Loewen, J. (1988). Visitation fatherhood. In Bronstein (Ed.), *Fatherhood today: Men's changing role in the family*. New York: Wiley.

Madanes, C. (1981). *Strategic family therapy*. San Francisco: Jossey-Bass.

Madanes, C. (1984). *Behind the one-way mirror*. San Francisco: Jossey-Bass.

Madanes, C. (1990). *Sex, love and violence*. New York: Norton.

Madanes, C. (1991). Personal communication.

Mahoney, M., & Mahoney, K. (1976). Treatment of obesity: A clinical observation. In Williams et al. (Eds.), *Obesity: Behavioral approaches to dietary management*. New York: Brunner/ Mazel.

Minuchin, S. (1974). *Families and family therapy*. Cambridge, MA: Harvard University Press.

Minuchin, S., & Fishman, C. (1981). *Family therapy techniques*. Cambridge, MA: Harvard University Press.

Minuchin, S., & Nichols, M. (1993). *Family healing*. New York: Free Press.

Mittelmann, B. (1958). Analysis of reciprocal neurotic patterns of family relationships. In V. Eisenstein (Ed.), *Neurotic interaction in marriage*. London: Tavistock.

Parke, R. D., & Sawin, D. (1976). The father's role in infancy. *The Family Coordinator, 25*, 365–371.

Radin, N. (1981). The role of the father in cognitive, academic and intellectual development. In M. E. Lamb (Ed.), *The role of the father in child development*. New York: Wiley.

Radin, N. (1983). Increased father participation and child development outcomes. In M. E. Lamb (Ed.), *Fatherhood and family policy*. Hillsdale, NJ: Erlbaum.

Richman, J. (1978). Fatherhood: The social construction of pregnancy and birth. In J. Richman (Ed.), *The place of birth*. New York: Oxford.

Schiff, N., & Belson, R. (1988). The Ghandi technique. *Journal of Marital and Family Therapy*.

Seltzer, J. (1991). Relationships between fathers and children who live apart: The father's role after separation. *Journal of Marriage and the Family, 53*, 79–101.

Stanton, D., & Todd, T. (1982). Family therapy of addiction. New York: Guilford.

Tylor, E. B. (1865). *Researches into the early history of mankind* (pp. 287–297). London.

Wallerstein, J., & Kelly, J. (1980a). *Surviving the breakup: How children and parents cope with divorce.* New York: Basic Books.

Wallerstein, J., & Kelly, J. (1980b). Effects of divorce on the visiting father-child relationship. *American Journal of Psychiatry, 137*, 1534–1539.

Watzlawick, P., Bavelas, J., & Jackson, D. (1967). *Pragmatics of human communication.* New York: Norton.

David R. Grove, who is in private practice at The Westerville Family Consultation Center in Columbus, Ohio, is also an adjunctive faulty member at the Ohio State University College of Social Work, and provides consultation and training for several agencies throughout Ohio. A supervisory member of the American Association for Marriage and Family Therapy, he has served as a member of the regional faculty for the Family Therapy Institute, D.C. In addition to publishing numerous articles on family therapy, Grove coauthored *Conversations on Therapy* with Jay Haley.

Rhonda Burnaugh is a registered nurse who has served the mental health community for more than 25 years. She has worked in inpatient as well as outpatient settings, with both adults and children. Burnaugh has a particular gift for helping severely disturbed clients by approaching them in nonmedical, empathic ways.